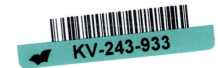
MEASURING HEALTH:
A PRACTICAL APPROACH

Edited by

George Teeling Smith

Director, Office of Health Economics
London, UK

A Wiley Medical Publication

JOHN WILEY & SONS
Chichester · New York · Brisbane · Toronto · Singapore

Distributed in the United States of America, Canada and
Japan by Alan R. Liss Inc., 41 East 11th Street, New York,
NY 10003, USA.

British Library Cataloguing in Publication Data:

Measuring health : a practical approach.
  1. Health status indicators
  I. Teeling Smith, George
  613   RA407

ISBN 0 471 91849 0

Printed and bound in Great Britain.

MEASURING HEALTH:
A PRACTICAL APPROACH

Contents

List of Contributors   vii

Foreword   ix
Professor Sir John Butterfield

1   Introduction   1
George Teeling Smith

2   Measuring Health in Clinical Care and Clinical Trials   7
Sonja Hunt

3   The Development of Health   23
Paul Kind

4   Techniques of Health Status Measurement using a Health Index   45
Gillian Capewell

5   The Time Trade-off Approach to Health State Valuation   69
Martin Buxton and Joy Ashby

6   Assessment of Quality of Life in Parkinson's Disease   89
Peter Welburn and Stuart Walker

7   Assessment of Treatment in Cancer   109
H. Schipper and J. Clinch

8   Assessment of Treatment in Rheumatoid Arthritis   157
Morton Paterson

9   Assessment of Treatment in Heart Disease   191
Bernie O'Brien

10   Assessment of Treatment of Irritable Bowel Syndrome   211
Jane Stevens, Jeffrey Poston and Stuart Walker

11   Applications in Management   225
Alan Williams

12   Implications for Clinical Practice   245
Colin Roberts

Index   263

List of Contributors

J. ASHBY
Health Economics Research Group, Brunel University, Uxbridge, UK

M. BUXTON
Health Economics Research Group, Brunel University, Uxbridge, UK

G. CAPEWELL
Formerly at Office of Health Economics, London, UK

J. CLINCH
Research and Planning Directorate, Manitoba Health, Winnipeg, Canada

S. M. HUNT
Research Unit in Health and Behavioural Change, University of Edinburgh, Edinburgh, UK

P. KIND
Centre for Health Economics, University of York, York, UK

B. O'BRIEN
Health Economics Research Group, Brunel University, Uxbridge, UK

M. PATERSON
Smith Kline and French Laboratories, Philadelphia, USA

J. W. POSTON
Welsh School of Pharmacy, UWIST, Cardiff, UK

C. ROBERTS
University of Wales College of Medicine, Cardiff, UK

H. SCHIPPER
Manitoba Cancer Treatment and Research Foundation, Oncology Unit, St Boniface Hospital, Winnipeg, Canada

J. C. STEVENS
Welsh School of Pharmacy, UWIST, Cardiff, UK

G. TEELING SMITH
Director, Office of Health Economics, London, UK

S. R. WALKER
Centre for Medicines Research, Carshalton, Surrey, UK

P. WELBURN
Senior Research Project Manager, Janssen Pharmaceutical Ltd, UK

A. WILLIAMS
Department of Economics, University of York, York, UK

Foreword

In Britain, the tax-payer pays the lion's share of the national bill for medicines through the tax-supported NHS.

There can be no doubt that the supplier of this long list of compounds, new and old, the pharmaceutical industry, gets a bad press. I am personally persuaded that this is at least in part because today's newspaper, radio and television producers, researchers, newscasters and programme people are generally young, attractive and healthy. Compared with older people, they have been well protected from illness and consequently have little appreciation of the contribution medicines now make to the quality of life of so many of our citizens. Doctors, whatever the public may be guided to think, are convinced about the therapeutic revolution and prescribe these very powerful substances and vigorously defend their rights to do so under their clinical freedom.

In the end, the catastrophic side-effects of a very small number—less than a score out of the thousands of compounds provided under the NHS—have themselves had some good side-effects. They have resulted in a drive to develop measures aimed at assessing the quality of life as part of clinical trials of new treatments. So an important by-product has also been the growing interest in assessing *health*, rather than *disease*. For far too long, doctors have been accused by their rivals in the market place—homoeopathists, acupuncturists and so on—of being completely dominated by the concepts of disease and treating patients with potentially dangerous chemically derived medicines. Indeed, this sort of idea has spilled over as a criticism of medical training programmes currently in use. I still get plenty of letters and remarks about the so-called but reviled 'medical model', which seems to be a belief that doctors *do* regard their patients as cases of diseases and categorize them as so, and then treat them by computer-directed regimens—a sad reflection of the profession's willingness to accept modern technology and start to record clinical details in easily accessed computer data-banks!

So it is very apt that just at the moment Professor George Teeling Smith and his expert colleagues got together and now publish their discussions about how health professions can measure *health*, which is what the patients and their relatives naturally have become primarily interested in, now that we can treat effectively so many diseases which were masters of our bodies and fates in the recent past.

I therefore hope that this book will be very widely read, very widely discussed and that it will stimulate more work in this important field. I hope too that the dear public reader will recognize what it is all about—part of our reaching up for the best in medicine, therapeutics and health promotion generally.

PROFESSOR SIR JOHN BUTTERFIELD

Measuring Health: A Practical Approach
Edited by G. Teeling Smith
© 1988 John Wiley & Sons Ltd

1

Introduction

George Teeling Smith
Office of Health Economics, London

This book is subtitled 'a practical approach' to measuring health. This might suggest that the techniques are already well established, and the methods of measurement are now straightforward. However, this is far from being the case. As some of the subsequent chapters will demonstrate, much research is still needed to produce universally accepted and validated methods to measure the 'quality of life' of patients before and after medical or surgical treatment. Nevertheless, pharmaceutical companies, medical research workers and doctors as a whole should already be becoming aware of the importance of measuring 'health' in social and economic terms as well as in narrowly defined clinical terms. The traditional approach of recording 'symptoms' alone is rapidly giving way to the measurement of patients' well-being in much more broadly defined terms. How well can patients function in society? How contented are they? How full a life can they live? These, of course, are questions which have always concerned doctors and pharmaceutical manufacturers. However, the new development in the late 1980s is that these questions are now being asked in quantitative rather than purely qualitative terms. That is what this book is all about.

As has already been indicated, the methods and techniques are still being developed. At present their application is largely experimental. In many cases steps taken to measure a patient's 'quality of life' may be as much an attempt to validate the techniques of measurement as an attempt to demonstrate the extent of success from a particular treatment.

Certainly in many cases—for example heart transplants—the improvement in quality of life is so dramatic that any one of a variety of techniques of measurement will easily demonstrate the benefit of the operation. However, in more marginal treatments, it is still often the method of measuring health rather than the treatment itself which is 'at fault' if no improvement is measured. Over the next decade or two other techniques of measuring health will be continuously refined; but in the meantime existing techniques are already being used, and this book describes these techniques and their practical applications. It will become clear to the reader, however, that some of the measurements which are made using the existing techniques still need to be interpreted with caution. But medical researchers who are unaware of the developments which are going on in this field could easily find themselves at a serious disadvantage when others are already using the techniques, and contributing positively to their development. That is the importance of this book.

First, however, it is useful to look back over the history of the evaluation of medicines and surgical techniques, in order to see how and why the present position has been reached. Up to the 1930s, doctors relied primarily on 'clinical impressions'. If a form of treatment *appeared* to benefit some patients it was accepted as being of value. These early clinical impressions as we now know, could be seriously misleading. The practices of 'cupping' and bleeding patients have long since been abandoned as doing more harm than good. But in the nineteenth century they were judged to be valuable forms of therapy. Similarly, in the pharmacoepia, strychnine and arsenic featured prominently and were widely prescribed. These too, have fallen by the wayside as doctors have learnt to mistrust their earlier 'clinical impressions'.

By the 1950s, for medicines at least, the principle of the randomized controlled clinical trial had become established as the only reliable way to assess the medical outcome of a new treatment. Gradually, the same principle is being applied to surgery. There have been some classic trials of well-established operations, such as the complete removal of a breast for a localized cancer, which have resulted in new attitudes to surgical practice. No pharmaceutical can now be marketed without substantial evidence of its efficacy and relative safety based on well conducted clinical trials. The same approach is becoming widely accepted amongst surgeons. Thus the traditional reliance on clinical impressions has given way to dependence on controlled clinical trial evaluation.

The next stage in the assessment of medicines and surgery came in the 1960s, when the principle of 'cost-benefit-analysis' was introduced by early health economists. These studies attempted to demonstrate that clinically successful treatments could sometimes also pay off in economic terms. A typical early example was in the control of tuberculosis. The first publication from the Office of Health Economics in 1962, *Progress against Tuberculosis*, showed that the 'conquest' of tuberculosis saved an amount equal to half the total cost of all medicines prescribed for all diseases under the British National Health Service. More recently, a publication by Teeling Smith and Wells in the *Pharmaceutical Journal* (10 August 1985), has shown that the hospital savings through better treatment of just nine diseases resulted in savings which exceeded the cost of *all* Health Service medicines by over £400m in 1982. Thus, it is still often possible to show not only clinical but also financial benefits from the use of modern medicines.

However, medical, social and economic changes have been taking place over the past ten years or so which mean that these traditional measures of the 'success' of treatment are no longer always relevant. For example, in the 1960s calculation on tuberculosis, much of the saving came from a reduction in absence from work due to sickness. Since the 1960s, however, two new factors have arisen. The first is unemployment; often if a person is made fit for work they will merely swell the numbers of unemployed. There is, therefore, no economic saving. Furthermore, although it is possible to show a dramatic reduction in sickness absence for an individual disease, total absence attributed to sickness has been rising in all western countries. People now feel more able to take time off work for relatively trivial ailments. Hence, on a global scale, the changing attitudes to sickness and to work have been associated with an economic loss rather than an economic gain.

There has been an equally dramatic effect as a result of the changing pattern of mortality. Again, in the 1960s, tuberculosis was typical, in that it killed young adults—as did lobar pneumonia and other infectious diseases. Thus a reduction in mortality from these causes added to the numbers in the productive working population. In the 1980s, by contrast, death from disease typically occurs in the older age group. With heart disease, for example, most deaths occur during retirement. If these deaths are postponed, the survivors *add* to the burden of dependency in society, rather than lightening it.

Thus the economic arguments of the 1960s are often now irrelevant. Successful therapy in many cases reduces the average national wealth rather than increasing it. However, it is obvious that *well-being* as opposed to wealth is considerably increased by reducing sickness and extending longevity. Thus economists have faced the challenge of quantifying this increase in well-being by measuring the 'quality of life' in addition to measuring its length. It can be argued, of course, that health is only one of many factors which affect a person's quality of life. However, the fact that at present health has been singled out for attention in this context in no way reduces the importance or validity of measuring health-related well-being.

More generally, the World Health Organization has for many years been advancing the idea that 'health' should be more broadly defined than merely the 'absence of disease'. WHO has advocated that good health should be represented by complete physical, mental and social well-being. That is, 'official' thinking has moved a long way away from measuring 'health' as something which one quantifies with a clinical thermometer or a sphynomanometer. Health concerns the whole person, and their relationship with the society in which they live. This, again, lies behind the new approach to measuring the state of a person's health by measuring their quality of life in the health context.

In more practical terms. the measurement of quality of life has become increasingly important because of the present fashion for cost-containment in health services. It has become much more essential to demonstrate quantifiable improvements in well-being in order to justify the cost of achieving it. But even more important, it has become essential to quantify the benefits of therapy in order to set them against the inevitable risks of modern treatments. Mere clinical measurements or anecdotal evidence that patients 'feel better' has not been sufficient to contradict the belief that a particular treatment is 'too dangerous' to remain in use. There needs, in the late 1980s, to be a formal benefit-risk equation in order to balance the human hazards of a medicine against its previously unquantified social benefits. If such equations had been available in quantitative terms it is quite possible that some treatments which have been withdrawn from the market could still be available to be prescribed in suitable cases.

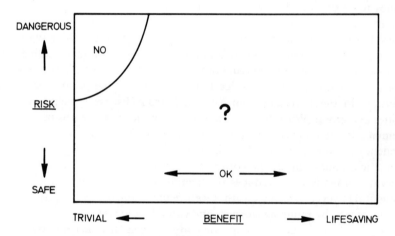

Figure 1. Teeling Smith Risk-Benefit Matrix

In this context, the 'Teeling Smith Risk-Benefit Matrix' is relevant. It is illustrated in Figure 1. One axis shows the relative risk of a treatment, and the other the relative benefits. If the risks are negligible, the treatment is acceptable however trivial its benefits. If its risks are severe, they are only justifiable if the benefits are dramatic—for example, a lifesaving treatment for cancer or AIDS. What is self-evident is that serious risks are never justified if the benefits are trivial. However, an important aspect of this risk-benefit matrix is that a treatment may shift its position both according to the type of patient being treated and according to the national economic situation.

Chloramphenicol is a good example. It has grave risks, but these are fully justified in treating typhoid. In this case, the product is in the top right hand corner of the matrix. But if it is used in western society to treat a mild sore throat, it shifts across to the top left hand side. And when it comes to the poorest countries of the world, its use is more justified (because of its cheapness) in moderately severe conditions than it would be in western societies which can afford much more expensive but safer alternatives.

That digression nicely illustrates the subjective nature of 'acceptable' benefits. But it also underlines the importance of the measurements themselves. Without some hard quantification of both risks and benefits, judgements on the acceptability or otherwise of a medicine must be based on pure speculation or prejudice.

Thus in the 1980s it is possible to make a convincing case for the importance of measuring the 'quality of life'. What will become clear in succeeding chapters is that there is still some uncertainty on exactly how such measures should be obtained.

As the subsequent chapters explain, the techniques can be divided broadly into the use of 'health profiles' or 'health indices'. There is also an important development with the use of the so-called 'time trade-off' technique, which requires patients to judge how long a period in one state of health could be 'traded' for a different period in another state of health. Obviously, the better their state of health, the shorter period of life people would accept as a 'trade-off' for longer survival in a less desirable state.

The problem is that simple 'health indices' based on peoples' subjective assessment of the relative values of different states of health can give results which vary from those using the 'time trade-off' method. Indeed, the indices themselves can be calculated in different ways. Meantime, therefore, most of the studies reported in this book rely on the simpler concept of a health profile—which will be fully described in later chapters.

However, the present uncertainties in the state of development of the measurement of health should not be allowed to cloud the principal issue. Classical cost-benefit analysis and simple measurement of medical signs and symptoms are no longer sufficient in themselves always to justify the choice of a new treatment.

What matters in the last decades of the twentieth century is how the patient *feels*, and not what the doctors think he 'ought' to feel, based on clinical measurements alone. This is an important development in medical philosophy, and one which is being steadily accepted by the medical profession. It will not, of course, be universally understood in the immediate future. The principle of the randomized clinical trial took many years to gain acceptance. However, the important point is that 'measurement of health' will become a generally accepted concept by the twenty-first century, and those who want to learn more quickly about the way in which the relevant techniques are being developed will gain much by reading this book. This is the justification for calling it 'a practical approach'. The techniques it describes may not always be immediately applicable or fully validated, but physicians and others concerned to be at the leading edge of developments in medical care will find much of practical relevance in its pages.

Measuring Health: A Practical Approach
Edited by G. Teeling Smith
© 1988 John Wiley & Sons Ltd

2

Measuring Health in Clinical Care and Clinical Trials

Sonja Hunt
Research Unit in Health and Behavioural Change, Edinburgh

The measurement of health is inextricably linked to two associated issues: how 'health' is defined and the purpose for which measurement is designed.

Definitions of Health

Exactly what is meant by the term 'health' can often only be inferred from the way in which the term is used. A decline in overall mortality rates in a population may lead some writers to conclude that 'health' is improving; the fact that one drug induces fewer side effects than another may be used to imply that the former is better for 'health' than the latter. Since in order to measure something it is vital to know what that something consists of, any consideration of health measurement must begin by dispelling, as far as possible, the semantic confusion which bedevils the term 'health'.

There is, unfortunately, little general agreement on definitions of health and attempts at clarification have ranged from suggesting the mere absence of discernible pathology to an all-encompassing focus on 'physical, social and mental well-being' (WHO, 1978). For the purposes of measurement, however, it is possible to gain some operational guidelines by breaking concepts of health into four categories each of which implies a different focus for measurement.

Disease

Disease refers to a biomedical nomenclature which reflects the interest and responsibilities of the medical profession. The diagnosis of a disease involves a

7

labelling process orientated to the problems of treatment and research where the underlying components of the process are largely incomprehensible to the lay person. Diseases may be discerned by reference to symptoms and clinical signs and, increasingly, the armamentarium of diagnostic technology. The assessment of the presence of disease is, obviously, a task for the medical practitioner, but the incidence and prevalence of disease in a population may be measured by reference to mortality and morbidity data.

Illness

Illness, on the other hand, may be defined as the experience of some distress or discomfort based upon an individual's perception that some change has occurred in customary function and/or feeling. The perception of illness is a subjective process with idiosyncratic elements and is usually relative to a background of 'noise'—that is, little aches and pains, slight malfunctions, feelings of unease, to which the individual has become accustomed. A person may feel ill, but not have a disease, or conversely may come to attract a medical diagnosis without feeling ill, for example in many cases of hypertension. The language of illness is that of the vernacular and is orientated towards problems of existence and coping which are of concern to the patient. The measurement of illness, therefore, must be orientated towards the patients' point of view, and will involve the use of interviews and questionnaires.

Sickness

Sickness is generally taken to refer to socially sanctioned ways of indicating illness, including acts of labelling and communication of distress. It involves a variety of behaviours including, perhaps, the seeking of medical attention, absence from work, staying in bed and the relinquishing of usual social activities. Neither illness nor disease necessarily implies sickness and, of course, sickness behaviour may be observed in the absence of either illness or disease. Measuring sickness may involve utilization rates of various medical specialties, or the assessment of sickness/absence rates.

Health

Both lay and medical personnel find it difficult to identify the definition and components of health except by reference to the absence of disease, illness and sickness. Moreover, the term 'healthy' sometimes implies some moral or value judgement as in the term 'a healthy attitude' which complicates the issue further. Health, in the positive sense is difficult, if not impossible, to measure by virtue of the fact that insufficient agreement exists on the components of health. Clinical judgements focus upon the presence or absence of disease, while lay people may hold a variety of concepts, such as the ability to carry out normal everyday tasks, having reservoirs of strength, feeling good, having the capacity for wholehearted enjoyment of life, being physically fit and so on (Herzlich, 1973; Hunt and MacLeod, 1987). In any event, the basic material upon which to base scales of reliable measurement is not currently available.

Related to the term health are others such as 'well-being' and the increasingly ubiquitous 'quality of life'. It is probably best to regard all these terms as hypothetical constructs which may be defined and operationalized for specific purposes. The confusion which surrounds definitions of health is an important one from the point of view of measurement since it accounts for the diversity of content and emphasis of the variety of so-called health indicators. The ambiguity of some health measures is attested to by the fact that the same instrument may turn up under rather different rubrics, for example, the Nottingham Health Profile, which is described later, has been referred to as an indicator of health status, a quality of life instrument and a measure of perceived distress.

The Purpose of Measurement

Clearly, the reason for measurement being deemed necessary is closely related to the variables that are to be measured. The extent and pattern of diseases in a population, for example, is important for the understanding of the overall impact of medical services, public health activities and social and economic conditions on health. This will require studies of an epidemiological nature, which may, of course, also be of value in assessing the aetiological significance of certain factors.

At the clinical level, the purpose of measurement may be to gain information about the pre-treatment status of the patient, which may have implications for both the choice of treatment and the outcome of that treatment; to assess the relative efficacy of various forms of therapeutic intervention; to measure the impact of treatment upon the patient, rather than upon the disease; to monitor post-treatment progress; to compare individual and group responses to different forms of treatment.

Doctor–Patient Discrepancies in the Assessment of Interventions

Medical care and treatment have proceeded almost since their inception without the apparent need for health measures which go beyond the judgement of clinical signs and symptoms. The previous chapter has indicated some of the reasons for the increasing popularity of health or quality of life measures. In recent years research has been carried out which indicates that discrepancies exist between the judgements of doctors and patients on whether some medical intervention has been efficacious or not. One of the best known studies is that carried out by Jachuck *et al.* (1982) on 75 hypertensive patients and their relatives. The authors found that in the opinion of the doctor concerned, all the patients had improved after treatment. However, less than half the patients shared this opinion and none of their relatives, all of whom thought the patient had deteriorated or remained unchanged. These discrepancies are easily explained once it is realized that each group based their judgement upon different criteria of 'improvement'. From the physician's point of view blood pressure had been satisfactorily controlled, there had been no clinical deterioration and the patient had not complained. The patients were judging in relation to their previous feelings, their ability to function and by their enjoyment of life. Relatives had noticed irritability, mood changes, lethargy and hypochondria, as well as deterioration in sexual energy and activity.

Similarly, in a study of outpatients in a general medicine clinic there was only 50 per cent concordance in doctor–patient assessments of the success of treatments (Orth-Gomer *et al.*, 1979). Research on low back pain has shown even less agreement on whether therapy has provided relief (Thomas and Lyttle, 1980). Moreover, doctors' assumptions about clinical symptoms which they feel ought to be associated with adverse effects on well-being are known not to be always correct. For example, in a comparison of cytotoxic and endocrine treatment for breast cancer. it was found that nausea, vomiting, constipation and total alopecia were more frequent in women on cytotoxic drugs. However, this was not reflected in their feelings of well-being which actually rose over an eleven week period (Priestman, 1986). It was concluded that the symptomatic relief resulting from tumour shrinkage more than offset the distress from side effects. In another study of quality of life following heart transplantation, Lough *et al.* (1985) observed that although heart transplant patients experience recurring symptoms and distress this has little impact upon their subjective evaluation of their overall quality of life.

Relatively few indicators have attempted to measure or even record the perception of the individual in relation to improvement and/or disability and yet we are coming to understand that it is these subjective elements which are largely responsible for whether or not an individual seeks care and considers himself/herself to be well. The relationship between 'objective' and 'subjective' is often regarded as a methodological problem, yet it may be more useful to regard the two aspects as being essential to our knowledge of human beings and their reactions—the one view enriching the other.

The need to incorporate the perspective of the patient into clinical assessments, both of the impact of the medical condition and the sequelae of treatment, has manifested itself in many guises. Most often, the patient's rating of their feelings, functioning and/or symptoms is elicited via some form of questionnaire, but the resulting information may be referred to variously, as indicative of 'quality of life', 'well-being', 'socio-medical data', 'perceived health status', or whatever term happens to be current. In reality most of the questionnaires do not measure any of the above, but rather focus upon aspects of disability, discomfort and distress. Concepts such as 'quality of life' and well-being, not only, to date, defy measurement because of lack of definition, but are so closely bound to the hopes, fears, values and expectations of individuals as to be unsuitable for making judgements about groups of patients or indeed about any patient in particular.

On the other hand, the fact that most questionnaires focus upon the negative aspects of function and experience is quite practical, since there tends to be a greater commonality in relation to that which is distressing, for example, pain, trouble with sleeping, sexual difficulties, than in respect of those experiences which enhance the quality of any individual life. The aggregation of scores thus becomes less problematic.

Comparisons of value in health-related activities must allow the perceptions of the patient an equal, if not greater, place than clinical evaluations. The patient's subjective assessment may elicit more practical interpretations of the meaning of the impact disease and treatment have on comfort whereas 'objective' indicators may merely be projections of professional mores. On the other hand, such measures will lack power if they are not convincing in the eyes of clinicians, technicians, manufacturers of drugs and equipment, whose orientation is towards 'hard data'. Health measures must be acceptable to those on both sides of the intervention at issue, for their capacity to enlighten the investigators and their appeal and appropriateness for patients.

Types of Health Measurement

Health measurements relevant to clinical concerns take several different forms according to the definition adopted, the purpose for which they are being used and the prejudices of the compilers. Thus a common type of measure takes the form of a list of symptoms to which the patient is asked to respond in terms of affirmation of varying degrees. Such measures express clinical concerns with the disease implications of signs and symptoms such as breathlessness, pain, cough, unusual bleeding, the production of sputum, bowel function and so on.

Attempts to introduce areas of more concern to patients are represented by functional measures such as the Sickness Impact Profile (Bergner *et al.*, 1976; 1981) adapted for use in Britain as the Functional Limitation Profile (Patrick, 1981). The SIP consists of 136 items which refer to illness or disease-related dysfunction in 12 domains including work, leisure, home life, mobility and social interaction. It thus measures, as its name implies, the impact and limitations on normal daily functions which are of most interest to the patient. Obviously, the underlying notion here is that a person's satisfaction with life and the quality of that life is impaired by interference with function.

Another type of indicator which reflects a lay perspective of health problems is the Nottingham Health Profile (Hunt *et al.*, 1986). This is a short 38-item questionnaire couched in the vernacular, which taps felt distress in the areas of physical mobility, pain, sleep, social isolation, emotional reactions and energy. The main advantage of this Profile is its brevity and its acceptability to patients. Within the six sections items have been weighted based upon lay judgements of the relative severity of the different experiences implied by the items.

Use of Health Measures in Clinical Care

The majority of medical practitioners probably think of health or quality of life as equivalent to normal functioning or as close to it as can be achieved under the circumstances. The correction of some medical condition may, therefore, satisfy the doctor, but for the patient other factors may have equivalent or greater importance, for example, concerns with family, work or leisure pursuits. Moreover, some criteria of function which may be used by the doctor to assess recovery, ignore other aspects of life. For example, one study showed that return to work following myocardial infarction was at the expense of other activities, leisure pursuits and sex life in particular (Finlayson and McEwen, 1977).

The treatment of mild or moderate hypertension provides a good example of the need for some adjunct to clinical outcomes. It is becoming well known that many antihypertensive therapies have side effects. Cognitive impairment, memory lapses, anxiety, sleep dysfunction, and impotence have all been reported (Bulpitt, 1982; Pickering, 1974). These effects are disturbing enough but their repercussions for the totality of the patient's life may not be appreciated. The ability to carry out occupational tasks may be impaired and income threatened. Feelings of tiredness may lead to lowered productivity and loss of interest, which is noted by employers. Personal relationships may suffer and be further disrupted by the irritability of the patient. For the sexually active, interference with customary enjoyment will have implications for harmonious and intimate relationships and for self-image. Often a patient may not associate these effects with medication and believe problems at work or in the home to be the fault of colleagues and family and sleep disturbances to be due to worry.

For some patients the ability to lead what they consider to be a normal satisfying life may outweigh any possible benefits of medication. Effects on daily life are a primary cause of lack of compliance to medical regimens. A study by Dunnel and Cartwright (1972) indicated that 16 per cent of pre-scribed items are thrown away before being used and 20 per cent of medicines are not taken as directed. In all only about 50 per cent of patients comply with doctors' advice and treatment. Non-compliance may be quite logical from the patient's point of view; feeling better, the occurrence of unexpected and unexplained side-effects or signs of drug toxicity are all good reasons for dis-continuing treatment. Solutions to non-compliance tend to be seen in improved doctor–patient communication and education. Conrad (1985) has described the alternative patient-centred approach to managing medications and points out that what appears to be non-compliance from a medical perspective may actually represent an attempt by the patient to assert control over his or her own disorder.

This emphasis on mutual decision-making would seem to indicate the value of including a shared outcome measure of perceived health as the basis for reviewing therapeutic intervention. Moreover, patients are often reluctant to discuss details of their life outside the surgery or clinic with the doctor and some means of assessing function and feelings which go beyond a cursory enquiry about the presenting condition can be of great value.

A further application of patient-based measures is in groups of patients where there is considerable uncertainty of prognosis. Cancer patients are an example of such a group. Individuals or certain categories of patients may be at higher risk of psychological disturbance in the early stages of clinical treatment and therefore might benefit from specialized care and support. In addition, in the longer term, questionnaires can assist in monitoring progress and add an additional perspective to clinical assessments, which might help to inform the direction of further therapy. The special problems of toxicity and side effects associated with cytotoxic therapy have been noted by Priestman (1986) especially where this is used following surgical treatment to treat possible micrometastasis. He described two measures which give accurate and sensitive assessments of measuring subjective toxicity but considered that, although these may give an indication of quality of life, further refinement was needed. A preliminary study of the use of the Nottingham Health Profile illustrated this approach with cancer patients (Hunt *et al.*, 1986). Of new patients attending for radiotherapy it was found that approximately 20 per cent experienced little or no evidence of distress as measured by the NHP. The remaining 80 per cent had poor subjective health status with some of the highest levels of distress possible, especially in emotional reactions, lack of energy and sleep. There appeared to be a relationship between perceived health at diagnosis and at the end of therapy, with those with the worst problems at diagnosis showing little improvement after treatment.

Patients with skin cancer showed least distress in perceived health at time of diagnosis and there was a considerable improvement following treatment. The data suggested that diagnosis engenders a great deal of emotional distress, particularly in females, but much of this has dissipated by the start of treatment. In a group of patients with residual or recurrent disease there were lower levels of perceived discomfort and distress than with new patients, but poor perceived health in the domains of sleep and energy for men and emotional reactions and social isolation for women. There also appeared to be more disability in daily life although this may reflect the fact that they formed an older age group.

In a small group of patients who were attending for follow-up and who had no residual disease the scores were fairly low. In all categories of cancer patients there was a considerable range in scores on the NHP, with some individuals having high or very high scores. Such analyses may allow individuals with special needs to be detected and within each disease grouping extra support can be given to those with the greatest expressed problems. This may allow extra help to be given to those who do not complain as well as those who are more vocal in expressing their problems. Molleman *et al.* (1984) indicated the importance of expert help in providing information and in assisting the patient and his or her close relative in reducing anxiety.

A further use of patient self-assessment is in the possible prediction of problems which do not show up on clinical examination. A study of pregnant women, monitored through the period of their pregnancy, showed that scores on a standard measure of perceived health problems, particularly in relation to social isolation, a lack of energy, sleep disturbance and emotional upset, were associated with future medical and social complications (Hunt *et al.*, 1986).

A deterioration in a patient's condition, or indeed an improvement, does not always manifest itself in clinical signs. Although most doctors listen to the comments and complaints of patients, they tend to do so with a clinical ear, alert for issues of medical not psychosocial concern. The inclusion of health or 'quality of life' questionnaires in assessments of clinical intervention has often been a rather cavalier affair. It is common for such instruments to be included because they are available, rather than because they are suitable for the particular circumstances. In fact, if the results obtained are to be of any practical value health measures must be chosen very carefully and used with understanding of their applicability, reliability and limitations. Some clinicians may have an interest in and understanding of the importance of including an assessment from the patient's perspective, but do not know what to measure, how to measure or how to judge the applicability, usefulness and merits or otherwise of particular instruments.

The choice of a health measure for use as an adjunct to clinical assessment will be optimized where the following factors are taken into account.

The Relevance of the Measure to the Medical Condition and the Treatment

This involves consideration of the main impact of the health problems and the probable effects of treatment. For example, there would be no point in using an instrument like the Sickness Impact Profile if the outcomes were likely to have little effect on function, but rather more likely to have an impact on intellectual ability.

The Reliability and Validity of the Instruments

For a questionnaire to give consistent results relevant to the issue under measurement it should have undergone extensive testing for reliability and validity and most reputable instruments will be accompanied by details of this. Reliability is normally established by a test/retest method and is, of course, closely related to the sensitivity and specificity of the instrument. In general it can be said that the less severe the items contained in the questionnaire the less consistent will be the results obtained with it. This is because more severe items tend to be more stable and robust.

Validity testing will take the form of running the instrument in trials of its relationship to other criteria which can be supposed to be indicative of the same underlying concept. In the case of the Nottingham Health Profile, for example, scores on the questionnaire were compared in relation to utilization of medical services, on the assumption that those who manifested greater distress through scores on the Profile would also be likely to seek medical attention. The discriminative power of the scores was tested by comparing those from groups with very different medical conditions and by before and after studies of medical intervention (Hunt *et al.*, 1986).

Very often questionnaires used in clinical situations have not been sufficiently tested for reliability and validity, often representing a set of ideas incompletely conceptualized and arbitrarily expressed. Most technical equipment in medicine has undergone a prolonged period of testing in order to ensure that it gives consistent and appropriate results. If the addition of questionnaires and interviews which tap the patients' view of medical intervention are to be taken seriously they must, equally, inspire confidence in the quality of their performance.

Previous History of the Instrument

It is important to know with which types of groups the instrument has previously been used and with what result. Is information available about its applicability to certain categories? For example, a study of the effects of chemotherapy on female cancer patients will clearly give a different pattern of scores than would one on men with moderate hypertension. It is helpful if comparison scores are available, particularly if a health measure is to be used only once with one group of patients. Clearly a 'quality of life' profile of, say, angina patients is of little value if there is no way of knowing how their scores compare with 'normal' individuals of the same age and sex. Since social class is also known to affect health experience (Hunt *et al.*, 1985) some information on this will always be helpful.

The Sensitivity to Changes Implied by a Particular Treatment

There is little point in including a health measure in clinical assessment if it is unlikely to pick up the probable effects of treatment. For example, some drugs may improve a patient's functioning but make them feel irritable, antisocial and depressed. Equally, some drugs may improve mood, but adversely affect gait and sleep. Clearly, judicious choice of instruments is necessary in order neither to over- nor to underestimate the value of the treatment and its impact on non-clinical aspects of the patient's life.

Acceptability to the Patient

This issue involves the language in which questions are couched, the time taken to complete the questionnaire and the kinds of items that are present. The average reading age of the British population is nine years. One of the major problems with health questionnaires which are devised by medical and health personnel is that the items they contain may be expressed in terms which are not completely understood by patients. This leads to misunderstandings and invalidates any results obtained. The actual content of the questionnaire must make sense to the patient and be seen as having relevance to his or her situation.

The burden imposed on the patient in terms of the time and patience required to fill out a questionnaire is an important consideration, particularly if he or she is seriously ill. A huge battery of instruments such as that employed, for example, by Croog *et al*. (1986) in the clinical trial of antihypertensive drugs not only affects compliance but constitutes a tiring, time-consuming task which may be taxing for the respondent. Another aspect of acceptability concerns the characteristics of the patient group. A self-administered questionnaire may pose practical problems for elderly persons who may find it difficult to hold a pencil because of arthritic fingers or who may have mislaid their spectacles.

Who Will Code and Analyse the Questionnaires?

Lengthy questionnaires with complex scoring systems may require specially trained coders and analysts. If such are not available, the simplicity of a questionnaire should be taken into account when deciding between equally suitable alternatives.

In summary, when choosing a health or 'quality of life' measure to be included either in clinical assessment of individual treatment or in a big trial, the reliability, validity, acceptability and comparability are of prime importance. If such measures and the information derived from them are to be taken seriously at least as much thought should be given to their choice as to the choice of treatment.

Use of Health Measures in Clinical Trials

The usual form of a clinical trial is that it is prospective and involves the random assignment of patients to different treatment groups, one or more of which will be a control. Eligibility criteria and details of the intervention to be tested are clearly specified and there is prior identification of primary and secondary outcomes. The samples involved will be of sufficient size to permit the application of statistics to the data and to allow conclusions to be drawn about significant differences between groups. Ideally, such a study is double blind.

The introduction of patient assessment of outcome into such a design poses a great many problems for the investigators, for the patients and for the reliability of the data. Probably of prime importance is the seriousness with which questionnaires are regarded by the personnel involved in that trial. Van Dam *et al.* (1981) have shown that non-cooperation of clinicians is the biggest barrier to organizing research in a clinical setting. Marks on a piece of paper may be perceived as of little value compared with the familiar clinical signs. Often staff do not appreciate the extensive testing procedure that standard questionnairies have been through and they need to be convinced both of the 'respectability' of the instrument and of the reason for its inclusion. Where this is not the case, administration of the questionnaire may become lax or even omitted altogether if staff are 'too busy'. Obviously, in a clinical trial variability in administration will lead to results which are of equivocal worth.

The consistency of administration of questionnaires, the location where they are filled in and who else is present, will also affect comparability of data. Although some personnel may not know who is on which drug, where questionnaires are given at regular intervals in the presence of the same staff member it may become apparent, through the pattern of responses, to which treatment group the patient belongs.

The setting in which questionnaires are given needs careful thought. A busy outpatient clinic is not the ideal location. If the instrument is filled in at home other family members may influence the answers. Whichever setting is chosen, subsequent administrations must be given in the same place; this requirement in itself may determine the location.

The time available for the completion of a health measure will influence the choice of instrument. In a hospital situation it may be possible to leave a self-assessment form with the patient for a longer period of time than in a clinic. The length of the questionnaire may also influence compliance with filling it out. Some trials, for example that reported by Croog *et al.* (1961), have used a whole battery of 'quality of life' measures involving a weighty series of questionnaires which imposes a heavy burden on patients as well as posing serious questions about the continuing reliability of the data. The frequency with which a questionnaire is given can affect the conclusions drawn from it. Where repeat applications are necessary too infrequent an administration will mean that transient effects are missed, but too frequent presentation may lead to contamination of one set of answers by the previous one and to increased attrition due to the imposition of the task on the patient's time and tolerance.

The seriousness with which patients regard a questionnaire is also of vital importance for compliance, although with well tried questionnaires this will have been established in the development phase. Nevertheless, the reason for inclusion of a health measure, its rationale and importance should always be explained. Too often questionnaires are handed to the patient in an off-hand manner which conveys the message that its completion is not a serious matter. Questionnaires should always be checked for the comprehensiveness of their completion as soon as they have been obtained from the patient; leaving them to pile up before checking may allow errors and omissions to multiply.

All of these issues are magnified when multicentre trials are in progress, since there may be substantial variability in the circumstances of administration of the questionnaires and the attitudes of the research team. Since the wider psychosocial aspects of health status are susceptible to influences outside the intervention at issue it is necessary to be aware that participation in the trial may itself have an effect on patients' well-being, and for this reason changes in treatment groups and placebo groups should always be compared with any changes in a control group and with comparison scores if available. Experimental groups may also be affected by increased attention or better nursing care.

Providing that these difficulties are recognized and systematically addressed health measures provide a useful, and sometimes decisive, independent outcome assessment and may well be crucial in the selection of alternative therapies when clinical outcomes are very similar or inconclusive.

One aspect of using randomized controlled trials to assess the impact of medical intervention is that important information concerning the interaction of the patient with the treatment may be lost in the aggregation of data. Because perceived distress and discomfort are somewhat related to unique factors in a patient's life and the context and meaning of that life, in a way that clinical indicators are not, the impact of the same intervention may be very different for different patients, a fact which may be obliviated by summary results.

The inclusion of some measurement of the impact of treatment on the wider aspects of a patient's experience is an ethical, as well as a practical, necessity when the testing of a new drug or treatment is being planned. The decision to apply a new therapeutic technique requires an appreciation of the total impact it may have, not solely the biomedical effects. A lowered mortality risk in exchange for an impoverished and difficult life may not be congenial to many people and a desired outcome of clinical trials must be the limitation, preferably the elimination of undesirable side-effects.

Cross-cultural Issues

An increasing number of clinical trials involve sites in more than one country. When this is the case the issue of comparability of health measures in different languages arises. Too often, some existing measure in, say, English, is chosen, simply translated in arbitrary fashion into the new language and used. This procedure is totally inadequate and there are a number of steps which must be followed systematically if there is to be the same degree of confidence in the translated instrument as there is in the original. Full details of the problems of cross-cultural adaptation have been given elsewhere (Hunt, 1986) but at a minimum the following procedures need to be employed:

the obtaining of multiple translations based upon thorough discussion of conceptual and semantic nuances of the items;

back translation into the original language and comparison of the two versions;

choice of the most acceptable version with substitution and/or omission of unsuitable items;

the presentation of the chosen translated items to a panel of lay people who will judge their acceptability and face validity.

Often at this stage it is found that some of the translations are not 'natural' to common speech and are expressed in language which is too literary. After the resolution of such problems a first draft of the translated questionnaire should be prepared and tested in the field on representative samples of patients. At this stage more problems of acceptability may arise and must be corrected.

After a final version has been agreed upon the questionnaire must undergo reliability and validity testing in the new culture and, if items in the questionnaire are weighted, a retrial of the weighting must be carried out.

Where this has been done it has been found that cultural values may affect the seriousness with which some types of distress and discomfort are regarded and it is to be expected that there will be differences between countries (Hunt and Wiklund, 1987). These procedures can take a year or more, but it is essential to follow them if the data obtained from the translated version are to be of any worth. Often there will be pressure to avoid or attenuate this process because of time constraints. However, there is little point in going to a great deal of administrative trouble to include a measure if the data obtained from it can be justifiably disregarded. Moreover, lack of time indicates lack of forethought and does not auger well for the smooth running and scientific rigour of the research.

Conclusion

Even a modest effect of treatment regimens on a patient's lifestyle and well-being raises important issues, especially when the outcome of treatment is uncertain. In recent years much progress has been made in the development and testing of health measures which can assess reliably the impact of medical intervention from the patient's point of view. Such measures are becoming increasingly robust scientifically and are of particular validity in that they raise and address issues fundamental to the function of medicine—the maximization of enjoyment and meaning of life even in the presence of illness. It is vital, however, that such instruments are used properly and taken seriously by clinicians, health personnel and patients alike.

References

Bergner, M., Bobbitt, R. A., Carter, W. and Gilson, B. (1981). The Sickness Impact Profile: development and final revision of a health status measure. *Medical Care*, **19**, 787–805.

Bulpitt, C. J. (1982). Quality of life in hypertensive patients. In Avery, A., Fagard, R., Lijnen, P. and Staessen, J. (eds), *Hypertensive Cardiovascular Disease: pathology and treatment*, The Hague: Martinus Nijhoff, pp. 929–48.

Conrad, P. (1985). The meaning of medications: another look at compliance. *Social Science and Medicine*, **20**, 29–37.

Croog, S. H., Levine, S. Testa, Marcia A., Brown, B. *et al.* (1986). The effects of antihypertensive therapy on quality of life. *New England Journal of Medicine*, **314**, 1657–64.

Dunnel, K. and Cartwright, A. (1972). *Medicine Takers, Prescribers and Hoarders*, London: Routledge & Kegan Paul.

Finlayson, A. and McEwan, J. (1977). *Coronary Heart Disease and Patterns of Living*, London: Croom Helm.

Herzlich, C. (1972). *Health and Illness: a social-psychological approach*, New York: Academic Press.

Hunt, Sonja M. (1986). Cross-cultural issues in the use of socio-medical indicators, *Health Policy*, **6**, 149–58.

Hunt, Sonja M., McEwan, J. and McKenna, S. P. (1985). Social inequalities and perceived health. *Effective Health Care*, **2**, 151–60.

Hunt, Sonja M., McEwan, J. and McKenna, S. P. (1986). *Measuring Health Status*, London: Croom Helm.

Hunt, Sonja M. and Macleod, M. (1987). Health and behavioural change: some lay perspectives. *Community Medicine*, **9**, 68–76.

Hunt, Sonja M. and Wiklund, I. (1987). Cross-cultural variation in the weighting of health statements: a comparison of English and Swedish valuations. *Health Policy*, **8**, 227–235.

Jachuck, S. J., Brierley, H., Jachuck, S. and Willcox, P. M. (1982). The effect of hypotensive drugs on the quality of life. *Journal of the Royal College of General Practitioners*, **32**, 103–5.

Lough, M. E., Lindsey, A. M., Shinn, J. A. and Stotts, N. (1985). Life satisfaction following heart transplantation. *Journal of Heart Transplantation*, **IV**, 446–49.

Molleman, E., Krabbendam, P. J., Annyas, A. A. *et al.* (1984). The significance of the doctor–patient relationship in coping with cancer. *Social Science and Medicine*, **18**, 475–80.

Orth-Gomer, K., Britton, M. and Rehnqvist, N. (1979). Quality of care in an outpatient department: the patients view. *Social Science and Medicine*, **13A**, 347–51.

Patrick, D. (1981). Standardisation of comparative health status measures: using scales developed in America in an English-speaking country. In Sudman, S. (ed.), *Health Survey Research Methods: third biennial conference*, Hyattsville, Maryland.

Priestman, T. (1986). Measuring the quality of life during cancer therapy. *Update*, 1 June, 987–98.

Thomas, M. R. and Lyttle, D. (1980). Patient expectations about the success of treatment and reported relief from low back pain. *Journal of Psychosomatic Research*, **24**. 297–301.

Van Dam, F. S., Somers R. and Beck-Couzijn, A. L. (1981). Quality of life: some theoretical issues. *Journal of Clinical Pharmacology*, **21**, 1665–85.

World Health Organization (1978). *Definitions of Health*. From the Preamble to the Constitution of the WHO basic documents, 28th edn, Geneva, WHO, p.l.

Measuring Health: A Practical Approach
Edited by G. Teeling Smith
© 1988 John Wiley & Sons Ltd

3

The Development of Health Indices

Paul Kind
Centre for Health Economics, York

Background

The term 'measurement', in the physical sciences, often conveys the impression of a precise operation based on well-established procedures, carried out in controlled laboratory settings and producing results which are expressed in terms of standardized units of measure. This scenario contrasts markedly with the attempts of social scientists to develop measures of health status where not only is the phenomenon under investigation defined in many different ways, but there are varying opinions as to how it might be represented, and on whether it could or should be quantified. As a consequence there have been a number of distinct and largely uncoordinated efforts to develop measures of health status. This chapter describes some of the processes involved in constructing measures of health status, looking firstly at some of the methodological issues which are central to the development of these measures and then going on to describe how these issues have been dealt with in practice.

Health status indicators may be classified according to a number of characteristics, and a distinction is sometimes drawn between indicators on the basis of their format—single composite indexes and multidimensioned and irreducible profiles. The use of the term 'profile' or 'index' in the naming of some measures of health status can, however, be positively misleading. Consequently the term 'indicator' is taken here to refer generally to all forms of health status or quality of life measure, irrespective of their format, much of the methodology of health status measurement being, in any event, common to all types of indicator. An additional note on terminology should also be made at this point. The actual mechanisms used to record health status measurement, be they a questionnaire or physician-led interview or simply a checklist, are referred to here as measurement *instruments*. This does not imply that they possess any particular level of refinement or accuracy, or indeed that they are capable of expressing observations in a quantitative form, merely that they provide the means for capturing information on health status.

Mortality and Morbidity

At a time when infectious diseases were more commonplace and their ultimate outcome was often fatal, the use of mortality data would have been a reasonable proxy measure of health status in the population There have, however, been fundamental changes in patterns of disease and causes of death over the last 50 years and in developed western societies gains in life expectancy are now relatively small. Life expectancy for a 45-year-old male in England and Wales was 26.4 years in 1951, compared with 27.5 years in 1981; this increase is less than half that achieved in the first 30 years of this century. Nevertheless, in the absence of any more suitable measure, mortality data, expressed as standardized rates, have been used as a proxy for health status in the population and in determining the allocation of health care resources. Mortality data may be useful in making comparisons between population subgroups, or as indicators of public health, but they have limited value in providing information about individual patients.

Morbidity data, recorded as days lost through sickness or disability, may capture information on a range of factors besides health status, including the availability of health care resources and the attitudes of the 'ill' person towards health. Epidemiological data on disease incidence or prevalence are recorded in accordance with a standard international classification. Information of this type is sometimes difficult to interpret. Environmental factors, unrelated to the provision of health care services, such as weather conditions in winter, can profoundly alter the pattern of morbidity (or even death). Changes in diagnostic procedures or simply increased awareness amongst doctors and the community also contribute to the instability of these data. Where population health status is concerned it may be difficult to select diseases which are good markers for the purposes of comparison over time, or between populations. Mortality and morbidity data essentially categorize individuals in terms of a single event— death or illness. The health status of individuals in the first category is clear and generally speaking unequivocal. Where ill people are concerned, however, traditional indicators are not able to distinguish a gradation of health status, and they are silent, too, about comparisons between diseases or conditions— how, for example, does lung cancer 'score' relative to pneumonia?

Measuring health status is not in itself a recent phenomenon. Rosser (1983) attributes one of the earliest examples of a health status index to the ancient Babylonians, some 1800 years BC. The code of Hammurabi specifies the penalties and rewards for the surgeon in his treatment of the patient, and these can be used to deduce a rough scale of values for both successful and unsuccessful interventions. In the mid nineteenth century, Florence Nightingale devised a scheme for describing the health state of patients on discharge from hospital using a hierarchical classification system of three categories: 'relieved', 'unrelieved' and 'dead' (Rosser, 1983). Both cases embody the twin components (description—valuation) to be found in present-day health status indicators.

Description

In spite of the fragmented research effort in this field, and irrespective of the form or function of the eventual instrument, a common understanding of the problems of constructing a health status indicator has emerged. In order to measure health status we need first to *describe* it in such a way that different levels/states are identified. A descriptive system is required in order to make the simplest form of measurement possible, that is to establish a relationship between a subject (patient) and some point or level on a health status continuum. Such a descriptive system might be based on a conceptual model which expresses the researcher's personal views of the relevant and measurable aspects of health or upon an existing definition, for example that of the WHO, expressed in terms of social, emotional and physical well-being. No matter how the descriptive components of the indicator are specified, researchers are at this point effectively limiting the extent to which their instrument is practically capable of registering different aspects and levels of health status. Those elements which are not explicitly included in the descriptive system will not be fully represented and any subsequent efforts to weight the system may undervalue their contribution. This may be less of a problem where a fairly well-defined group of patients or a single disease process is involved, since the researchers are more likely to have an intimate knowledge of the condition and its impact on the patient. Where researchers adopt this 'top-down' approach and specify the elements of the descriptive system themselves, without reference to a wider set of judges, there can be no certainty that all *relevant* components have been included. Precisely what constitutes relevance, and who judges it are important considerations, in themselves.

The problem of designing a comprehensive descriptive system may be tackled in another way, so as partially to overcome the difficulty of judging what should be incorporated in the descriptions—namely, asking individuals to provide the material directly. Surveying the community, or a specific patient group, can yield large volumes of descriptive material about the effects of ill health on usual functioning and quality of life. These data might be expressed in terms of statements made by the individual respondents about themselves, or in more general terms about the effects of ill health on other people. This open-ended approach to constructing the descriptive base produces an almost endless stream of information and much of it may be fairly idiosyncratic, especially where the respondent is given the opportunity to speak about their own, or their family's experiences of ill health. Analysis of these data itself poses some awkward problems for the researcher. Faced with an abundance of data he has to find some way or organizing, refining and reducing it so as to produce a viable set of descriptions, preferably one in which the use of language is simple, non-technical and unambiguous, and which is compact enough to permit subsequent valuation. The processes involved in this 'bottom-up' approach are likely to be every bit as judgemental as those which characterize the prior specification of the 'top-down' strategy. Some of the researcher's ideas about how the descriptive material should be organized will inevitably influence the direction of the data analysis. Techniques such as multidimensional scaling or factor analysis which may produce statistically acceptable representation of the empirical data still require the researcher himself to make decisions about how the dimensions/factors are labelled or described.

Valuation

Although simple forms of measurement are possible using a descriptive system alone, its usefulness can be significantly enhanced by the addition of a valuation or scoring system which *quantifies* different levels of health status, thus permitting the magnitude of changes in health status to be observed and measured. Introduction of a valuation system raises additional problems however, and two issues in particular will have to be considered—*whose valuations should be sought*, and *how should these be derived*? The case might be argued for selecting ill people, as a group who perhaps have the most acute awareness of the effects of ill health, Similarly doctors and other health care professionals might be represented as having a broader and more objective view of the relative severity of health states—as the 'experts', they too should be consulted. Individuals in good health might be thought of as being more detached from the influences of training or experience and therefore capable of giving a less biased set of responses. Ultimately, of course, since decisions have to be taken about the allocation and use of health care resources, it might be thought appropriate that any weights which are to form part of a health status measure should originate with politicians and the government. The use of a single reference group for weighting a health status indicator is to be avoided unless the weights are only to be applied in the specific context of a single disease or condition. Multiple reference groups provide much needed information about the variability in scores which may arise from different subject groups.

While the construction of a soundly based scoring system is an important requirement in developing a useful indicator, not all researchers have been concerned with a detailed examination of the processes involved. In some instances the scoring system has been specified by the researchers themselves on the basis of an arbitrary weighting of their own design. A slightly less crude means of generating a scoring system for a descriptive health status indicator involves surveying a population sample to establish the frequencies with which different health states are encountered. These frequency data might then be converted into a simple numeric scale using one of a variety of models (e.g. Guttman). The scoring system might be so arranged that commonly occurring health states were given the highest weighting and the least common state, presumed to be the more serious, attracted lower weights.

Scaling Techniques

The analysis of attitudinal and subjective response data drawn from a variety of sources has a long and honourable tradition (e.g. Thurstone and Chave, 1929) which continues to the present day (e.g. Orth and Wegener, 1983). Stevens (1966) distinguishes between three types of scaling procedure which have been used for measuring non-physical stimuli comparable to health states, for example the seriousness of crime (Sellin and Wolfgang, 1964). *Magnitude estimation* is designed to elicit valuations directly from subjects. A single health state might be designated as a reference state by the experimenter and this would be assigned a unit value. The subject is asked to indicate the magnitude of the ratio between that reference state and other health states and to express this ratio as a number. If states B and C scored 4 and 8 respectively when compared to the reference state A (with its pre-assigned value of 1), then that subject's scale values for A, B and C would be taken as 1, 0.25 and 0.125. The geometric means or median scores for the experimental subject group should be used to represent the average valuations for each state. Where the rank order of states has been established prior to magnitude estimation then it is permissible to work with successive pairs of states, rather than continually making judgements with respect to the reference state.

Category rating, in one or other of its variants, forces subjects to classify states into one of a limited number of ordered categories. These categories are sometimes represented as being separated by equal intervals, although this is a difficult assumption to sustain. The typical rating scale will at least be bounded by descriptions of the end categories. Subjects are expected to sort the states into categories according to, say, their 'perceived seriousness'. The mean category score for each state can be calculated from the pooled experimental data. In its basic form this type of scaling, unlike magnitude estimation, does not support the examination of individual differences between subjects. Two variants of the procedure can assist in this, Rank ordering can be treated as a form of category rating in which the number of categories is equal to the number of health states. The mean rank sum based on the pooled responses can be used as scale values for the group as a whole and correlation coefficients (Spearman's rho) can be used to examine the association between subject rankings. Similarly, graphical rating procedures can be used to capture valuations. Ratings can be expressed on a visual analogue scale (often a 10 cm line), on which subjects record the point at which they consider a state should be located. ('unimportant'; 'extremely serious') or by a numeric value (0; 100). The scores for each state are obtained by simply measuring the distance along the line that has been marked by the subject.

Paired comparisons methods require subjects to make judgements about pairs of states, essentially answering the question 'is state A worse than state B?' No estimate is made of the magnitude of the relationship. Judgements about all pairs of states are required for the original model and this typically necessitates $n \times (n-1)/2$ judgements, although modifications to the procedure can circumvent this limitation where large numbers of states are involved. The analysis of paired comparisons data usually precludes the possibility of examining responses from individual subjects but measures of internal consistency are easily calculated and can be used to indicate the quality of the subjects' performance and the extent of any agreement amongst them.

The measurement level of any indicator should be carefully assessed in the course of its design and construction. Indicators which are published without proper evaluation of their measurement properties are likely to be limited in their usefulness and prone to misuse for purposes which they are intrinsically unable to support. In particular the arbitrary use of numbers to designate different levels within an indicator may lead to their spurious use as weights or valuations. Care should be exercised too, in the selection of the statistical tests which are used to analyse observations based on these indicators. Most forms of statistical analysis can be applied to data from interval or ratio scales which give rise to quantitative measurements (the arithmetic mean can legitimately be computed as a measure of central tendency, for example). Nominal and ordinal scales produce data which are essentially qualitative in character and should be subjected to non-parametric statistical tests (the mode or median would be the appropriate measure of central tendency in this case). If the theory and practice of scaling methods appears to be an unduly complex area of study the reader will find some reassurance in Torgerson's standard reference work on the subject (Torgerson, 1958).

Selecting a Scaling Method

The selection of the procedure for eliciting or generating valuations from subjects is crucial in two respects. Firstly, the scaling method which is adopted may require multiple ratings of health states and this can prove impractical for any but the smallest sets of descriptive systems. Individual subjects may not be able to complete more than one set of ratings without fatigue and consequent degradation in the reliability of their responses. Larger, more complex descriptive systems can be partitioned so that a single subject is exposed to only one segment for the purposes of collecting repeated ratings. This in turn calls for correspondingly larger numbers of subjects, so that sufficient judgements can be obtained for statistical analysis. The approach, however, seriously limits the opportunity for examining individual differences between subjects. A similar limitation holds if the scaling method aggregates judgements made by individual subjects, as with the method of paired comparisons. The single subject's preference matrix in this instance cannot be analysed using Thurstone's original model, although models which can cope with such data have been more recently described (Bradley and Terry, 1952). Categorical scaling methods have similar deficiencies.

The second consideration in selecting the scaling procedure is the measurement properties of the resultant scale. As has already been observed, the use of number is no guarantee of any arithmetic properties whatsoever in the final instrument. Their association with health states in some circumstances merely serves as a convenient labelling device. Some procedures give rise to scales with well-recognized measurement properties, although these cannot be automatically assumed, especially where the scaling process has been inadequately implemented or where the statistical analysis has been incomplete. Computing the relevant goodness-of-fit statistic can be a useful safeguard against incautious optimism. Violations of the theoretical assumptions upon which a scaling method is based should be critically assessed. A clear example of this can be seen in respect of the Nottingham Health Profile (McKenna *et al.*, 1981) which has been shown to be defective in the scaling of the Sleep category (Kind, 1982). Failure to attend to this detailed examination of the empirical data can only create additional problems in a research area already fraught with difficulty.

Since no standard measures exist against which the scoring systems of health status indicators can be validated, there is continuing controversy about the relative superiority of the various scaling techniques which have been employed and about the scale values which they produce. Scale values arrived at by different experimental procedures may or may not be in agreement. The selection of both scaling method and the form of the descriptive material has been shown to influence raters' responses (Llewellyn-Thomas *et al.*, 1984). The different measurements of temperature on Fahrenheit and Centigrade scales can be simply resolved and observations on one scale may be transformed into corresponding values on the alternate scale. Health status measurement has not yet reached the point where the relationship between different scales is so readily explained.

The first part of this chapter raised some of the methodological issues which can be encountered in the development of health status indicators. The second part reviews some examples of health status indicators which have been developed or applied over the past two decades of health services research.

The Functional Living Index-Cancer (FLIC) was developed to meet the need for an evaluative instrument which was capable of detecting changes in patients across a range of dimensions, not just physical well-being (Schipper *et al.*, 1984). It was designed specifically for use with cancer patients. The design of a questionnaire was entrusted to an 11-member panel which included patients, spouses of patients, physicians, nurses and a clergyman. An unspecified number of patient interviews were also conducted to establish important aspects of daily functioning—as seen by patients themselves. The panel considered the review and interview material before producing an initial 92-item version of the Index. Items which were too specific, or unclear, were eliminated following field testing. Subsequent validation exercises were conducted and with further refinement led to a final 22-item questionnaire.

The method of scoring this instrument is somewhat unusual. A scoring line, as used in visual analogue scales, is divided into seven categories and the patient records their response by making the point along the line which s/he feels best corresponds to their current state. Responses are then scored by taking the nearest category boundary to the visual analogue score. Scores for individual questions range from 1 to 7 and the overall value of the Index is produced by aggregating scores for each question. A score of 1, rather than zero, is assigned to what might otherwise be regarded as 'normal' or optimal responses. Although the scoring system is based on ordinal categories, and the ratings for questions appear to be aggregated across distinct dimensions, scores on the FLIC index are reported to be significantly correlated with scores recorded on the Karnofsky Performance Status Index as well as with measures of psychosocial function.

The QL-Index (Spitzer, 1981) is similarly a disease-specific indicator, again designed for use with cancer patients. Three panels of expert judges were used to draw up the descriptive material which forms the basis of this instrument. In this instance however, the content was derived exclusively from consultations with the panel. Items were selected from 'plausibly distinct groupings' which resulted from statistical analysis of panel responses. The Index comprises five dimensions: activity, daily living, health, support and outlook (see Table 1). There are three levels within each dimension and the patient is given a score of 0, 1 or 2 according to the assessment of the examining physician. The scoring system was designed along the lines of the Apgar scale (Apgar, 1953) and it is difficult to see how essentially ordinal categories can be combined to create a truly quantitative measure.

Both these specific indices were developed to meet a growing need for instrumentation which would aid in the evaluation of treatments within a single disease process. One index which is widely used as a quasi-generic measure of health status is the Karnofsky Performance Status Index which while originally designed for use in assessing patients with lung cancer (Karnofsky *et al.*, 1948), has been incorporated in a wide range of other settings. Originally devised as part of an evaluative study of the palliative treatment of lung cancer, the

Table 1. The Spitzer QL-Index

A score of 2, 1 or 0 is given according to the physician's assessment of the patient during the past week

Activity

2 Has been working or studying full time, or nearly so, in usual occupation; or managing own household; or participating in unpaid or voluntary activities, whether retired or not

1 Has been working or studying in usual occupation or managing own household or participating in unpaid or voluntary activities; but requiring major assistance or a significant reduction in hours worked or a sheltered situation or was on sick leave

0 Has not been working or studying in any capacity and not managed own household

Daily Living

2 Has been self-reliant in eating, washing, toiletting and dressing; using public transport or driving own car

1 Has been requiring assistance (another person or special equipment) for daily activities and transport but performing light tasks

0 Has not been managing personal care or light tasks and/or not leaving own home or institution at all

Health

2 Has been appearing to feel well or reporting feeling 'great' most of the time

1 Has been lacking energy or not feeling entirely 'up to par' more than just occasionally

0 Has been feeling very ill or 'lousy', seeming weak and washed out most of the time

Support

2 The patient has been having good relationships with others and receiving strong support from at least one family member and/or friend

1 Support received or perceived has been limited from family and friends and/or by the patient's condition

0 Support from family and friends occurred infrequently or only when absolutely necessary or patient was unconscious

Outlook

2 Has usually been appearing calm and positive in outlook, accepting and in control of personal circumstances

1 Has sometimes been troubled because not fully in control of personal circumstances or has been having periods of obvious anxiety or depression.

0 Has been seriously confused or very frightened or consistently anxious and depressed or unconscious

Index is an 11-point scale describing the extent of a patient's independence and his ability to carry out his normal activity (see Table 2). Each level is given a percentage score (100 = normal; 0 = dead), although these 'scores' are only notional values, written down by Karnofsky some 40 years ago. They were not the subject of any examination or inquiry at the time. Since its publication this Index has become embedded in the literature as perhaps the classic measure of its type. It is only more recently that the validity and reliability of the Index have been examined (Hutchinson *et al.*, 1979) and its status as a 'numeric scale'

Table 2. Karnofsky Performance Status Index

Definition	%	Criteria
Able to carry on normal No special care needed	100	Normal; no complaints; no evidence of disease
	90	Able to carry on normal activity; minor signs or symptoms of disease
	80	Normal activity with effort; some signs or symptoms of disease
Unable to work. Able to live at home, care for most personal needs	70	Cares for self. Unable to carry on normal activity or to do active work. A varying amount of assistance is needed
	60	Requires occasional assistance, but is able to care for most of his needs
	50	Requires considerable assistance and frequent medical care
Unable to care for self Requires equivalent of institutional or hospital care Disease may be progressing rapidly	40	Disabled; requires special care and assistance
	30	Severely disabled; hospitalization is indicated although death not imminent
	20	Very sick; hospitalization necessary; active supportive treatment necessary
	10	Moribund; fatal processes progressing rapidly
	0	Dead

has even now not been seriously challenged (Schag *et al.*, 1984, p.187). The Index has, as a result of this continued and largely uncritical acceptance, been used in a number of settings where its legitimacy must be seriously questioned, for example a study of bone marrow transplantation in children (Hinterberger *et al.*, 1987). Despite these shortcomings the Index does appear to have good prognostic properties—as an indicator of imminent death in the terminally ill (Evans and McCarthy, 1985).

The Barthel Index is of more recent vintage and was designed as a measure of independence in patients with neuromuscular or skeletal disorders (Mahoney and Barthel, 1965). It comprises ten categories which refer to aspects of daily activity including feeding, transferring from bed to chair, washing and bathing, dressing and control of bowels and bladder. Some categories are subdivided to give two or three levels, each one arbitrarily scored in increments of 5 points, for example, Feeding:

Score

10 Independent patient, can feed himself from tray or table when food within reach

5 Some help is necessary

The maximum score on the Index is 100 and indicates a patient who is continent, can dress, wash and feed himself, is able to get out of bed, able to negotiate stairs and can walk a short distance outside.

Grogono and Woodgate (1971) developed their Health Index with the intention of allowing severity of disease, efficacy and cost of treatment to be compared. The Index was based upon what they regarded as the usual activities of daily life. A 10-item questionnaire was designed for use by a doctor who scored his patient's responses 1, 0.5 or 0 depending on whether the patient was normal, impaired or incapacitated on each item. The total score for each patient was divided by 10 to produce the Health Index. Patients with a variety of complaints were assessed using this index and scores ranged from 0.25 for a case with severe asthma, to 0.95 for one with varicose veins. One interesting aspect of their paper was the suggestion that the Index could be used as a weighting factor to give a value in health terms to a period of time. A year in full health (1 'health-year') would be equivalent to two years with a Health Index of 0.5.

The indices which have so far been described are either highly specific to a single disease process or are restricted in their usefulness by virtue of a primitive scoring system which effectively makes them no more than descriptive instruments. Where more robust measurements are required, for example in quantifying rather than just observing changes in health status, then one of a limited number of 'indicators' might be considered. These general-purpose indicators were developed for use in a variety of different applications but all have

Table 3. Grogono and Woodgate's Health Index

---

1. Work: normal, impaired or reduced, prevented

2. Hobbies and recreation: normal, impaired or reduced, prevented

3. Is patient free from malaise, pain or suffering?

4. Is patient free from worry or unhappiness?

5. Does patient communicate satisfactorily?

6. Does patient sleep satisfactorily?

7. Is patient independent of others for acts of daily living?

8. Does patient eat and enjoy his food?

9. Is micturition and defaecation normal?

10. Has patient's state of health altered his sex life?

Patients score 0, 0.5 or 1 for their response to each of these 10 questions

---

attempted to establish a scoring system which reflects personal preferences and is based on responses from different groups of judges, not just the sometimes idiosyncratic views of the researcher.

Torrance *et al.* (1982) describes a health state classification system based on four attributes: physical function, role function, socio-emotional function and health problems (see Table 4). The system was devised as part of an evaluation of neonatal intensive care (Boyle *et al.*, 1983) and was considered capable of being used to classify the health status of children ages 2–15 years. A large number of health states are defined by this $6 \times 5 \times 4 \times 8$ descriptive system and the problems of scaling this volume of information were overcome using procedures which Torrance himself had developed (Torrance, 1976). The time trade-off method (TTO) is a technique which involves presenting the subject with the choice between a finite period of time in a chronic health state, and a shorter period of time in a healthy condition. The time in the second condition is varied until the subject is unable to distinguish between the two alternatives (a fuller account of the technique is presented elsewhere in this volume). The problem of scaling a classification of this type in which large numbers of states are defined is well known and various strategies have been put forward (Torgerson, 1958). While it is practical to consider having subjects make decisions about the ordering and weighting of levels *within* attributes or dimensions alone, it is beyond reasonable expectation to ask subjects to examine all possible combinations of levels *across* attributes. Multiattribute utility theory (MAUT, Keeney and Raiffa, 1976) offers a well-developed framework in which to resolve this problem. Each of Torrance's subjects was asked to rate levels within each of the attributes using a category scaling method. Time trade-off techniques were then used to establish the nature of the relationship between attributes.

By combining these experimental data according to MAUT rules it was possible to construct a function which assigns values to all of the 960 health states. A total of 112 subjects, parents of schoolchildren, took part in home interviews conducted by professional interviewers. Just under 80 per cent of the subjects produced acceptable data, defined as conforming to the experimenter's logical ordering of the attributes. The reader is referred to Torrance's original papers for a full account of the theoretical background and the specification of the multiattribute function which determines the values for health states in this classification system.

Table 4. Extract from Torrance's health state classification
(lower and upper categories for each dimension)

Physical function

Level 1   Being able to get around the house without help from another person; having no limitation in physical ability to lift, walk, run jump or bend

Level 6   Needing help from another person in order to get around the house; not being able to use or control arms and legs

Role function

Level 1   Being able to eat, dress, bathe and go to the toilet without help; having no limitations when playing, going to school, working or in other activities

Level 5   Needing help to eat, dress, bathe or go to the toilet; not being able to play, attend school or work

Socio-emotional function

Level 1   Being happy and relaxed most or all of the time and having an average number of friends and contacts with others
Level 4   Being anxious or depressed some or a good bit of the time, and having very few friends and little contact with others

Health problems

Level 1   Having no health problems
Level 8   Being blind or deaf or not able to speak

The McMaster Health Index Questionnaire (MHIQ) is the product of a multidisciplinary group, some of whom share past association with Torrance. The questionnaire was constructed following a review of existing instruments designed to measure social, emotional and physical function. In an early study (1977) the initial draft questionnaire was used by an interviewer to collect data on subjects in their own homes. The subjects' family doctors also completed a clinical assessment of their patients at about the same time, rating them in terms of function, and present and future health. Responses to the Index questionnaire were compared with the family doctors' observations and those items which demonstrated a good association were identified. These items were given scores according to their value in predicting the doctors' ratings. Similar analyses which examined the relationship between MHIQ questions and patients' self-assessment of health (Chambers *et al.*, 1978) were performed.

Although this chapter deals with health indices rather than with profiles there is a strong case for reviewing one profile here. The Sickness Impact Profile (SIP) collects information for scoring and presentation as either a profile *or* a single index. As a behaviourally based measure of sickness-related dysfunction it was designed specifically to incorporate lay-perceptions of sickness, not just those of professional care-givers (Bergner *et al.*, 1976). Groups of patients, health care professionals, individual carers and healthy subjects were asked to describe dysfunctional behaviour. As has already been noted, this approach is likely to generate a large and potentially endless stream of data. Some means of deciding a limit has to be instituted. A simple decision-rule in this study dictated that subjects continued to be recruited until the rate of new descriptive material fell markedly. Five research staff then reviewed the various statements obtained from the participants and worked independently to eliminate ambiguous statements. Some statements were rephrased so as to make them more explicit. The edited list of statements was then sorted, on the basis of their similarity, into groups.

The final version of the instrument consists of 136 statements covering 12 areas of activity of the type shown in Table 5. A two-stage procedure was adopted in scaling SIP. Firstly judges rated all statements *within* dimensions, using an 11-point category scale. Judges were given an opportunity to correct their ratings after completing each dimension. All judges rated each of the statements in all of the dimensions. The two statements which had been rated by judges as being the most and least dysfunctional within each dimension were subsequently rated by the same judges, this time on a single 15-point category scale, to enable comparisons between dimensions to be made. Subjects selected for the initial scaling of SIP included physicians, nurses and health administrators. Later replication of the scaling processes used subjects drawn from consumer groups. Valuations produced by the various groups, although separated by a two-year gap, were highly correlated.

Seven of the categories have been used to define major physical and psychosocial dimensions within the Profile. Respondents answer 'Yes' or 'No' to each statement and the corresponding item scores are used to construct a total for each of the 12 categories, an aggregate score for the two principal dimensions, or a global sum for the questionnaire as a whole. The validity and reliability of the Profile have been examined in some detail and the instrument has been used in a number of settings, including studies of the effects of early cardiac rehabilitation on quality of life (Ott *et al.*, 1983), and of patients with low back pain (Follick *et al.*, 1985). The SIP has been translated from its American

Table 5. Example statements from the Sickness Impact Profile

I do not walk at all (Ambulation)

I am staying in bed most of the time (Mobility)

I do not have control of my bowels (Body care)

I am sleeping or dozing most of the time (Social interactions)

I communicate mostly by gestures (Communication)

I have attempted suicide (Emotional behaviour)

I sometimes behave as if I were confused or disorientated in place or time (Alertness behaviour)

I am not doing heavy work around the house (Home management)

I am going out for entertainment less (Recreation and pastimes)

I am eating special or different food (Eating)

I sleep or nap during the day (Sleep and rest)

I am not working at all (Work)

---

setting and a recent paper (Patrick *et al.*, 1985) suggests that these efforts have been successful in converting both the language and the item weights. Such a development would open the way for exciting US/UK collaboration in the field of health status measurement.

Fanshel and Bush (1970), in their now classic paper, described a measurement model of health in terms of a function/disfunction continuum, along which a series of 12 function levels (health states) were ranged. Each state was to be weighted according to its position along the continuum. Bush and his co-workers sought subsequently to operationalize and develop this model. They considered that the potential number of descriptions of the function levels was 'almost limitless' and the composition of the function level description was finally identified by reviewing hundreds of cases reported in the medical literature, as well as items gleaned from survey instruments. The Quality of Well-Being Scale (Patrick *et al.*, 1976) consists of three ordinal scales on dimensions of daily activity: mobility, physical activity and social activity (see Table 6). Combinations of each scale were initially taken to define 29 function levels, each of which could be linked with a separate classification of symptoms and problems. A typical function level might be expressed as follows

Did not drive or had help to use bus (mobility)

Walked with physical limitations (physical activity)

Performed self-care activities but not work, school or housework (social activity)

Pain, stiffness or discomfort in chest. stomach, side, back or hips (symptom/problem)

Table 6. Function levels in the Quality of Well-Being Scale

Mobility	Physical activity	Social activity
Drove car and used bus or train without help	Walked without physical problems	Did work, school or housework and other activities
Did not drive or had help to use bus or train	Walked with physical limitations	Did work, school or housework but other activities limited
In house	Moved own wheelchair without help	Limited in amount or kind of work, school or housework
In hospital	In bed or chair	Performed self-care but not work, school or housework
In special care unit		Had help with self-care

A subset of 400 descriptions was selected from a much larger universe defined by the 29 function levels, 42 symptom/problem complexes and five age groups. Two groups of nurses and graduate students used a 16-point category scale to rate items drawn from this subset. Subsequent modification has increased the number of function levels to 43 and reduced the symptom/problem complexes to 21. Further groups of judges have been recruited to repeat the scaling using both category rating and magnitude estimation procedures. The Quality of Well-Being scale, in its current form, is an observer-completed instrument which requires an interview of between 10 and 15 minutes and is typically obtained by taking the average score for a 4-day period. It has been used in a number of evaluative studies screening PKU (Bush *et al.*, 1973), chronic obstructive pulmonary disease (Toevs *et al.*, 1984) and in drug trials (Bombardier *et al.*, 1986).

Rosser initially developed a set of descriptions of state of illness for use in measuring hospital output (Rosser and Watts, 1972). Doctors were asked to consider what information they used to assess the severity of illness in their patients. They were instructed to ignore prognosis or any information which might relate to a patient's future state of health. Two descriptive dimensions emerged following these discussions—disability or objective dysfunction and distress. Eight levels of disability and four levels of distress were defined in Rosser's descriptive system and combinations of these disability and distress levels were used to describe a total of 29 states of illness (see Table 7). For the purposes of this classification it was considered that an unconscious individual would not experience distress. The reliability and comprehensiveness of this classification was tested satisfactorily in a number of London Teaching Hospitals (Rosser and Watts, 1972; Benson, 1978). While the disability/distress states proved useful in describing the *distribution* of patients' health status they were unable at that stage to provide information about the magnitude of *changes* in health status which might be detected. Psychometric scaling methods were used to elicit valuations for the 29 states. Seventy subjects with different current experiences of illness, including medical and psychiatric patients, doctors, nurses and healthy volunteers, took part in structured interviews during which they were asked to rank a small subset of 6 'marker' states drawn from the full range of disability/distress descriptions. The relative severity of successive pairs of 'marker' states was estimated by the subject, and these ratio judgements were used to construct a rough numeric framework into which the subject placed the remaining states. When the subject had satisfactorily ranked and scored the 29 disability/distress states they were asked to assign a zero score to that state to which it would be reasonable to restore any ill person. Subjects were also required to locate death as a state within this set of valuations.

Variation in the valuations accorded to the health states was mainly attributable to the subjects' current experience of health. Medical and psychi-

Table 7. Rosser's descriptions of illness states

Disability

I	No disability
II	Slight social disability
III	Severe social disability and/or slight impairment of performance at work. Able to do all housework except very heavy tasks
IV	Choice or work or performance at work very severely limited. Housewives and old people able to do light housework only but able to go out shopping
V	Unable to undertake any paid employment. Unable to continue any education. Old people confined to home except for escorted outings and short walks and unable to do shopping. Housewives able only to perform a few simple tasks
VI	Confined to chair or to wheel chair or able to move around in the home only with support from an assistant
VII	Confined to bed
VIII	Unconscious

Distress

A	No distress
B	Mild
C	Moderate
D	Severe

atric patients produced significantly different scores. Both sets of patients, by contrast, closely matched the valuations of their respective groups of nurses. No significant differences were found when subjects were classified in terms of age, sex, social class or past history of serious illness (Rosser and Kind, 1978). The valuations were later transformed (Kind *et al.*, 1982) so that the least dysfunctional state scored 1 and death scored 0.

The Rosser disability/distress scale has been incorporated in patient studies in psychotherapy, chronic obstructive airways disease and end-stage renal failure. The scale has also been used alongside an established measure of neurological state in patients with traumatic head injury, and as a comparative instrument with the Nottingham Health Profile in a study of patients with intracranial disease. This measure has played an important part in the calculation of quality-adjusted life years (QALYs), described, for example. in an evaluation of coronary artery by-pass surgery (Williams, 1985) and in the analysis of clinical data to inform decisions about resource allocation (Gudex, 1986).

Summary

Health status indicators can be constructed as specific measures for use within a single condition or disease group, or as generic measures where wider, cross-diagnostic use is envisaged. The basic elements in the construction of a generic health status measure are fairly well-established—setting up a descriptive system which defines levels or states and then constructing a set of weights which quantifies the relationship between the states so that health status can be represented as a single index value. This latter process is common also to the construction of health profiles which differ from indices in that they are not usually capable of reduction by aggregating scores across categories or dimensions.

Important methodological questions are central to the construction of any health status index. The researcher may elect to utilize his own conceptual thinking when designing states or levels, without making reference to other groups of judges. Alternatively, he may devise a descriptive system based on material collected from a variety of sources. Whichever course of action is followed the researcher can influence the way in which health status is portrayed. This influence may extend to any subsequent weighting of the index by limiting the range of responses which raters can make.

Where a weighted generic health status index is being developed the choice of method used for valuing the descriptions of health status is also important since this will determine the arithmetic properties of the resultant scale. Different scaling methods give rise to different scales and in the absence of any 'gold-standard' with which to make comparisons it cannot be reasonably claimed that any one method is superior to the rest, although it may have technical advantages in its actual use. The relationship between scales produced by the various techniques currently in use is not fully understood and there is scope for systematic comparisons in this area of health services research.

The process of describing health states and of placing valuations upon them involves recruiting judges/raters and the selection of these participants will also influence the final outcome. The extent to which systematic variations exist in the perception of health by different subject groups has yet to be definitively researched. Where significant differences are found between subject groups then additional problems will be encountered in establishing a single representative aggregate weighting system. Since many of these methodological questions wait to be finally resolved, researchers who seek to measure health status within their own studies would be well advised to consider carefully the implications of these issues before embarking on the construction of a new instrument. Better still they might consider using a battery of existing measures with at least one generic index selected from the examples described here, and thereby contribute to a greater understanding of the practical problems of health status measurement.

References

Apgar, V. (1953). A proposal for a new method of evaluation of the newborn infant. *Current Researches in Anesthesia and Analgesia*, **32**, 260–7.

Benson, T. J. R. (1978). Classification of disability and distress by wardnurses: a reliability study. *International Journal of Epidemiology*, **7**, 359–61.

Bergner, M., Bobbitt, R. A. *et al.* (1976). The Sickness Impact Profile: conceptual formulation and methodology for the development of a health status measure. *International Journal of Health Services*, **6**(2), 393–415.

Bombardier, C., Ware, J. *et al.* (1986). Auranofin therapy and quality of life in patients with rheumatoid arthritis. *American Journal of Medicine*, **81**, 565–78.

Boyle, M. H., Torrance, G. W. *et al.* (1983). Economic evaluation of neonatal intensive care of very-low-birthweight infants. *New England Journal of Medicine*, **308**, 1330–7.

Bradley, R. A. and Terry, M. E. (1952). Rank analysis of incomplete block design. I. The method of paired comparisons. *Biometrika*, **39**, 324–45.

Bush, J. W., Chen, M. M. and Patrick, D. L. (1973). Cost-effectiveness using a health status index: analysis of the New York State PKU screening program using a health status index. In Berg, R. (ed.) *Health status indexes*, Hospital Research and Educational Trust, pp. 172–208.

Chambers, L. W., Segovia, J. *et al.* (1978). Indexes of Health: Lay and professional perspectives of physical, social and emotional. Paper presented at Sociology of Health Care conference, London, Ontario, May 1978.

Evans, C. and McCarthy, M. (1985). Prognostic uncertainty in terminal care: can the Karnofsky Index help? *Lancet*, 25 May, 1204–6.

Fanshel, S. and Bush, J. W. (1970). A health status index and its application to health services outcomes. *Operations Research*, **18**, 1021–66.

Follick, M. J., Smith, T. W. and Ahern, D. K. (1985). The Sickness Impact Profile: a global measure of disability in chronic low back pain. *Pain*, **21**, 67–76

Grogono, A. W. and Woodgate, D. J. (1971). Index for measuring health. *Lancet*, 1024–6.

Gudex, C. (1986). QALYs and their use by the Health Service. Centre for *Health Economics Discussion Paper 26*, York University.

Hinterberger, W., Gadner, N. *et al.* (1987). Survival and quality of life in 23 patients with severe aplastic anaemia treated with BMT. *Blut*, **54**, 137–46.

Hutchinson, T. A., Boyd N. F. and Feinstein, A. R. (1979). Scientific problems in clinical scales as demonstrated in the Karnofsky index of performance status. *Journal of Chronic Diseases*, **32**, 661–6.

Karnofsky, D. A., Abenmann, W. H. *et al.* (1948). The use of nitrogen mustards in the palliative treatment of carcinoma. *Cancer*, November, 634–56.

Keeney, R. L. and Raiffa, H. (1976). *Decisions with mltiple objectives: preferences and value tradeoffs*. New York: Wiley.

Kind, P. (1982). A comparison of two models for scaling health indicators. *International Journal of Epidemiology*, **3**, 271–5.

Kind, P., Rosser, R. M. and Williams, A. (1982). Valuation of quality of life: some psychometric evidence. In *The Value of Life and Safety*, Jones-Lee, M. W. (ed), Geneva: North-Holland.

Livingston, M. G. and Livingston, H. M. (1985). The Glasgow assessment schedule: clinical and research assessment of head injury outcome. *International Rehabilitation Medicine*, **7**, 145–9.

Llewellyn-Thomas, H., Sutherland, H. J. *et al.* (1984). Describing health states: methodolic issues in obtaining values for health states. *Medical Care*, **22**, 543.

Mahoney, F. I. and Barthel, D. W. (1965). Functional evaluation: the Barthel Index. *Maryland Medical Journal*, **14**, 61–5.

McKenna, S. P., Hunt, S. M. and McEwen, J. (1981). Wreighting the seriousness of perceived health problems using Thurstone's method of paired comparisons. *International Journal of Epidemiology*, **10**(1), 93–7.

Orth, B. and Wegener, B. (1983). Scaling occupational prestige by magnitude estimation and category rating methods. *European Journal of Social Psychology*, **13**, 417–31.

Ott, C. R., Sivarjan, E. S. *et al.* (1983). A controlled randomized study of early cardiac rehabilitation: the Sickness Impact Profile as an assessment tool. *Heart Lung*, **12**, 162–70.

Patrick, D. L., Sittampalam, Y. *et al.* (1985). A cross-cultural comparison of health status values. *American Journal of Public Health*, **75**(12), 1402–7.

Rosser, R. M. (1983). A history of the development of health indices. In *Measuring the Social Benefits of Medicine*, George Teeling Smith (ed.), London: OHE.

Rosser. R. M. and Watts, V. (1972). The measurement of hospital output. *International Journal of Epidemiology*, **1**, 361–8.

Rosser, R. M. and Kind, P. (1978). A scale of valuations of states of illness: is there a social consensus? *International Journal of Epidemiology*, **7**, 347–58.

Sackett, D. L., Chambers, L. W. *et al.* (1977). The development and application of indices of health: general methods and a summary of results. *American Journal of Public Health*, **67**(5), 423–8.

Schag, C. C., Heinrich, R. L. and Ganz, P. A. (1984). Karnofsky performance status revisited: reliability, validity and guidelines. *Journal of Clinical Oncology*, **2**(3), 187–93.

Schippper, H., Clinch, J. *et al.* (1984). Measuring the quality of life of cancer patients: the Functional Living Index-Cancer: Development and Validation. *Journal of Clinical Oncology*, **2**(5), 472–83.

Sellin, T. and Wolfgang, M. (1964). *The measurement of delinquency*, New York: Wiley.

Spitzer, W. O., Dobson, A. J. *et al* (1981) Measuring the quality of life of cancer patients. *Journal of Chronic Diseases*, **34** 585–97.

Stevens, S. S. (1966). A metric for the social consensus. *Science*, **151** 530–41.

Thurstone, L. L. (1927). A law of comparative judgement. *Psychological Review*, **34**, 273–86.

Thurstone, L. L. and Chave, (1929). *The Measurement of Attitudes*, University of Chicago Press.

Toevs, C. D., Kaplan, R. M. and Atkins, C. J. (1984). The costs and effects of behavioural programs in chronic obstructive pulmonary disease. *Medical Care*, **22**(12), 1088–100.

Torgerson, W. S. (1958). *Theory and methods of scaling*. New York: John Wiley.

Torrance, G. W. (1976). Social preferences for health states: an empirical evaluation of three measurement techniques. *Socio-Economic Planning Sciences*, **10**, 129.

Torrance, G. W., Boyle, M. H. and Harwood, S. P. (1982). Application of multi-attributable utility theory to measure social preferences for health states. *Operations Research*, **30**, 1043 69.

Williams, A. H. (1985). Economics of coronary artery by-pass grafts. *British Medical Journal*, **291**, 6491, 326–9.

Measuring Health: A Practical Approach
Edited by G. Teeling Smith
© 1988 John Wiley & Sons Ltd

4

Techniques of Health Status Measurement using a Health Index

Gillian Capewell
Formerly at Office of Health Economics, London

Quantitative Valuation of the Health Improvement *per se*—Health Status Measurement

In the past much of the emphasis of economic appraisal of health care programmes has been on valuing costs, changes in health services and community resources and economic benefits. That is, because of difficulties in quantification and valuation, changes in health state *per se* have tended to be omitted. This suggests, quite wrongly, that economic appraisal is synonymous with the assessment of merely the financial aspects of health treatments.

More recently there has been a growing tendency among health care professionals, researchers and economists to recognize the need to develop ways to measure and quantify the change in health status itself resulting from a given health care activity. In pursuing this aim three main approaches have been developed: the first involves the use of *ad hoc* numerical scales, the second is the willingness to pay/receive approach and the third is through the use of utilities and QALYs.

Focusing on the first of these, the use of *ad hoc* numerical scales involves assessing the individual on a number of aspects of his/her health, assigning numerical scores to each assessment and adding up the scores. Grogono and Woodgate (1971) used this approach for their 'Index for Measuring Health'.

They identified ten dimensions of human functioning which reflected the aspects of life upon which medicine was expected to have an impact. (See Table 1). The scoring system used was to allocate 1, $\frac{1}{2}$ or 0 to each factor according to whether the patient was normal, impaired or incapacitated. The score at a particular point in time for each patient was taken as the sum of the scores across all ten dimensions and the total was then divided by 10 to yield a health index. The authors suggested their instrument could be used to evaluate the benefits derived from medical treatment for individuals, and to allocate resources in communities for treatment and research.

Table 1. Components of the
Grogono–Woodgate Index

1.	Work
2.	Recreation
3.	Physical suffering
4.	Mental suffering
5.	Communication
6.	Sleep
7.	Dependency on others
8.	Feeding
9.	Excretion
10.	Sexual activity

Although that was an ambitious proposal, this like other such indexes is essentially arbitrary and has several serious methodological problems.[*] Other examples of this approach to measuring health status include the Harris Index (1971), the Karnofosky Index (1949) and Spitzer's QL Index (1981). For application in economic appraisal these indexes could be used as a measure of effect in cost-effectiveness analysis (CEA).

Drawing on the work of Schelling (1968), Mishan (1971) developed the willingness to pay (WTP) approach, which is based firmly in modern welfare economics. That is not to say that the principle is uncontroversial, but it is a

---

[*] Culyer (1978) points out that there was no apparent awareness in the study that certain value judgements were being made, and once exposed, these would not be the value judgements that the authors would be likely to make. These are: (a) the judgement that the 'rate of substitution' of one dimension for another is constant, that is, a half-unit increase in one dimension can always be exactly offset by a given decrease in any other dimension; (b) the judgement that an increase in one dimension is always exactly offset by an identical decrease in any other dimension; (c) the judgement that a move from one index contour to another gives equal increments of health status.

clearly well-understood philosophical rational. It rests on the idea that individuals' valuations are reflected in what they would be willing to pay to receive certain benefits or avoid certain costs. (Pay is used here in the sense of what individuals are willing to forego or sacrifice and not just in the monetary sense.)

The approach can take several forms. One alternative involves the use of actual market decisions as a basis for making inferences about WTP. For example, in a widely cited study, Thaler and Rosen (1975) looked at wage premiums paid to persons in hazardous occupations in return for accepting identifiable risks. A second alternative entails the use of survey-based inferences of WTP. Acton (1973) used a direct survey procedure to determine how much people would be willing to pay for emergency coronary care services which reduced the probability that a heart attack victim would die as a direct consequence of the heart attack. The use of decision analysis, which provides a set of procedures for explicitly analysing complex decision problems and choices according to the expected utility principle, constitutes a third alternative.

Rosser and Watts (1972) measured what they described as the 'Willingness to Receive' (WTR), as determined by the amount of a court award for monetary compensation for injury. They analysed about 500 awards made by the high courts of Great Britain empirically to determine the relative value of health states based on monetary criteria. Both WTP and WTR provide a monetary value which can be used in cost-benefit analysis (CBA). However, in addition to the objections of principle, many practical problems encountered in this approach have lead to its infrequent use.

The third approach to measuring health status, pioneered by Torrance, is through the use of *utilities* and *QALYs*. It depends on the use of a cardinal scale in which the differences between the individual values along the scale can be compared in a meaningful way. An every day example of such a scale is the use of degrees Centigrade for temperature measurement. Thus Torrance (1984) describes *utilities* as 'cardinal values that are assigned to each health state on a scale that is established by assigning a value of 1.0 to being healthy and 0.0 to being dead. (This shall now be referred to as the dead-healthy scale.) The utility values reflect the quality of health states and allow morbidity and mortality improvements to be combined into a single weighted measure, QALYs gained.' To use his example, if a health care programme improves the health of individual A from a 0.50 utility to a 0.75 utility for one year and extends the life of individual B for one year in a 0.50 utility state, the total QALYs gained for that year would be 0.25 for individual A plus 0.50 for individual B, giving a total of 0.75.

The determination of numerical weights or utility values, as referred to above, is the focus of attention in this paper, the contents of which are based on the aforementioned paper by Torrance. In tackling this problem the analyst has a choice of three alternative methods: judgement, the use of suitable existing utility values published in the literature, or the use of measurement techniques to measure the values him/herself. Once established, these weights or utility values can be used in practice to measure the quality of life either at a point in time or over a period of years for a group of actual patients.

Alternative 1: Judgement

The use of judgement to estimate utility values is undoubtedly the simplest method and has two advantages in that it is relatively quick and cheap. The analyst himself may make a simple estimation or a more formal measurement may be based on the knowledge of a sample of experts who will allocate different utility values to different states of health.

The unavoidable subjectivity of the judgmental approach, however, makes it necessary to carry out sensitivity analysis in those studies in which this method is adopted. If the analysis shows that the conclusions of the study are relatively robust, that is, relatively insensitive to wide changes in the subjectively assessed utility values, then this approach may be considered adequate. However, if the conclusions are sensitive to changes in the utility values, it would be necessary to obtain more credible values by using an alternative technique.

Alternative 2: Use of Utility Values taken from the Literature

There are a growing number of studies in which utilities for certain health states have been measured and published. By way of example, for end stage renal failure patients Churchill *et al.* (1984) published utilities for haemodialysis, continuous ambulatory peritoneal dialysis (CAPD) and transplantation. On a utility scale ranging from 0.00 for death to 1.00 for perfect health, the mean utility for chronic haemodialysis for the 42 patients receiving the treatment at the time of interview was 0.57. Similarly, for the 17 CAPD patients it was also 0.57, and for the 14 transplanted patients the mean had a value of 0.80. Pliskin and co-workers (1980) reported utilities for two levels of angina pain: mild and severe. Taking a pain-free year as having a utility value of 1.0, the estimated value of a year with severe chest pain ranged from 0.42 to 1.00 (with a mean of 0.69 and a standard deviation among estimated values of 0.22) and the estimated value of a year with mild chest pain ranged from 0.74 to 1.00 (with a mean of 0.88 and a standard deviation among respondents of 0.10).

These and other existing values, taken from the literature[*] may be employed by other researchers. Caution is required, however, to ensure the health states measured in the original study match those of the new study. In addition, the subjects used in the measurement process in the original study must be

---

[*] See for example utilities for loss of speech due to laryngectomy reported by McNeil *et al.* (1981), utilities for cancer-related states reported by Llewellyn-Thomas *et al.* (1982) and Sutherland *et al.* (1983).

appropriate for the new study. And finally, the original study must have used valid methods of measurement.

Alternative 3: Measurement of the Utility Values

A third and more accurate way to acquire utility values is for the analyst to obtain the values him/herself using formalized measurement techniques. Four stages can be identified in such a measurement process and each is considered here in turn:

(i) Identification of health states for which utilities are required.
(ii) Preparation of health state descriptions.
(iii) Selection of subjects.
(iv) Use of utility measurement instrument.

Stage (i) Identification of Health States

In the first stage each unique possible health outcome which may be encountered in the study should be identified. Inevitably the number of different health states which may be established in this way depends on the nature of the study itself. In a study of neonatal intensive care for very-low-birth-weight infants (Boyle *et al.*, 1983) there were 960 distinct possible health states. [A classification of health states was developed to measure the health of survivors according to their physical function (six possible levels), role function (five levels), social and emotional function (four levels), and health problems (eight levels). Thus, there were $6 \times 5 \times 4 \times 8 = 960$ health states.] Whereas, by contrast, a demonstration application of a utility maximization model (Torrance *et al.*, 1973) involved the measurement of utilities for just 5 health states (home confinement under treatment for tuberculosis, home dialysis, hospital-based dialysis and kidney transplant) for use in the evaluation of three health care programmes: a programme for mass chest x-ray and tuberculin testing, a screening programme for the prevention of haemolytic disease of the newborn, and a kidney dialysis and transplantation programme.

Stage (ii) Preparation of Health State Descriptions

Once each unique possible health outcome has been identified, health state descriptions should be prepared to be presented to the subject and/or used by the analyst. As a starting point, health states should be described in functional as opposed to clinical terms. That is, the description should focus on how easy or difficult it is for a person in a particular health state to be able to function. A statement on the level of physical, emotional and social functioning is required. And, since the utility of a specific health state is affected by its duration and prognosis, these should also be specified either in the description itself or as part of the measurement process. For chronic states, the prognosis should be stated as no change until death and for temporary states it should be stated as no change until the end of the temporary duration specified, at which point the person returns to normal health. Finally, the description should include the age of onset for the state and specify whether or not the state has to be thought of as applying to the subject himself or to someone else.

Following identification of the health states and preparation of health state descriptions, the analyst has three possibilities for describing a health state to a subject. When the relevant health states for utility measurement are simply those of the patients themselves involved in the study, the individuals can provide a utility measurement for their own health state. At first sight it would seem unnecessary in this case to provide a health state description; however, to enable others to interpret the results health state descriptions may still be required.

This approach (i.e. the use of patient's own health state) was adopted in the aforementioned study by Churchill *et al.* (1984). Torrance forecasts a considerable future for this approach in clinical trials. Here the quality of life, as measured by utility scores, can be determined on each subject in each of the experimental and control groups at baseline and at each follow-up point. And/or by asking patients in the study to compare their state of health now with that on entry to the study, changes in utility scores can be measured directly.

However, in the case of a subject who is not in a particular health state, he/she must be asked to assess a given state based on description. For example, consultants and graduate students in nursing and health administration were used to assess different health states in an analysis of a phenylketonuria (PKU) screening programme (Bush *et al.*, 1973). Similarly McNeil *et al.* (1981) investigated the attitudes of 37 healthy volunteers, interviewing 12 firefighters and 25 middle and upper management executives to determine their preferences for longevity as against impairment of speech through cancer surgery.

The level of detail in the health state description varies greatly from one study to the next. In the study above relating to speech impairment subjects were presented with a written 'scenario' to obtain their attitudes towards the absence of normal speech for various periods of survival. In addition, a tape recording was played to respondents, to illustrate the speech capabilities of two patients who had undergone the operation, laryngectomy. By comparison, Patrick *et al.* (1973) used descriptions that included merely a few key words or phrases which highlighted the chief characteristics of the health states.

Torrance (1984) reports that comparison among different approaches suggests that sometimes utility values differ depending on the level of detail and sometimes they do not. Other investigations have focused on the problem of bias in the answer, as determined in the way the health state is described. Torrance's advice for measuring utilities on the general public is to use abbreviated descriptions to avoid cognitive overload, to supplement those with prior, more detailed, explanations of the key phrases used in the abbreviated descriptions, and to avoid the framing bias by wording the question in a balanced (positive and negative) manner.

The third possibility for describing health states, which is the appropriate approach when large numbers of health states are involved, is to use a 'Health State Classification System' (HSCS) that incorporates all states of interest. An HSCS is based on the concept that health status can be defined in terms of a number of attributes. Each attribute is divided into a number of mutually exclusive and collectively exhaustive levels. The specific combination of levels, one from each attribute, is taken to represent a unique health state. In this way an HSCS may generate a very large number of health states. For example, if there are ten different levels for each of three attributes, one thousand discrete health states will be defined.

Different health state classification systems have been developed by various analysts for various uses. Bush and his co-workers developed a system for general use with four attributes (mobility, physical function, social function and symptom problem complex) (Kaplan *et al.*, 1976), while Rosser (1976) developed a system with just two attributes, disability and distress, for application to inpatients. Wolfson *et al.* (1982) developed a system for application to stroke patients with ten attributes (dressing, bathing, continence, eating, transfer, wheelchair, ambulation, understanding, speech and mental status) and Torrance *et al.* (1982) developed a system for general use with four attributes (physical function, role function, social emotional function and health problem).

Stage (iii) Selection of Subjects

The selection of subjects or individuals whose utilities are to be measured is a controversial issue. Different studies have used different types of people. Some have investigated patients' preferences (Churchill *et al.*, 1984) on the grounds that they can best appreciate the implications of particular health states, others have used a random sample of the population on the premise that society's preferences should count as society's resources are being allocated, and others have investigated the preferences of health professionals on the grounds that they are more knowledgeable.

On deciding who should be asked, the purpose and viewpoint of the study inevitably plays an important role. Thus the patients themselves are the appropriate subjects to ask regarding the utility of their condition in clinical trials. Similarly, *informed* members of the public are appropriate subjects in a study conducted from the societal viewpoint. 'Informed' implies, however, that the subject has a good knowledge of what the specified health state is like. This immediately raises the question of how to describe a dysfunctional health state to a healthy individual who has no prior experience of the particular state? To some extent the problem is overcome by careful design (style and content) of the health state description and through the use of reliable and valid (to be described later) measurement techniques. Emerging evidence also suggests that different groups do not generally produce different results (Kaplan and Bush, 1982; Sackett and Torrance, 1978) and hence the problem may not be unduly significant.

Stage (iv) Use of Utility Measurements

Before considering some of the measurement techniques developed to date, it is useful to go back to distinguish between ordinal, cardinal and ratio scales. An ordinal scale is simply a rank ordering of health states, in order of their preference with ties allowed, and is sufficient merely for answering questions of the sort 'How does the outcome of intervention A compare with the outcome of intervention B?'

Cardinal scales may be interval or ratio. Measurement on an interval scale implies that the zero point and the numbers assigned to the entities are arbitrary, save that they order them (as in ordinal measurement) and keep the ratio of the interval between them the same. This kind of measure is akin to that used for measuring temperature in fahrenheit or centigrade and is required to answer questions of the type 'How much more effective is A than B?' However, individual scores—like individual temperature measurements—cannot be added up.

With a ratio scale the origin is not arbitrary (i.e. zero means none) and only the unit of measurement is arbitrary (e.g. length in millimetres, centimetres or metres). A ratio scale provides values which can be added up (as distances can), and which indicate meaningful ratios between measurements. They provide answers to questions of the form 'Proportionately how much better is A than B?'

An ordinal scale is clearly the simplest to obtain but it is rarely adequate for use in economic appraisal. In recent years most activity has focused on the development of techniques to produce interval scales and each of the measurement techniques considered here produces interval scales of utility. The rating scale technique, the standard gamble technique and the time trade-off technique are described in the next section.

The Rating Scale

A typical rating scale consists of a line drawn on a page with clearly defined end points such as 'Death, least desirable' at one end and 'Healthy, most desirable' at the other. The remaining health states are then located on the line between these two in order of their preference such that the intervals between the placements correspond to the differences in preference between the health states, as perceived by the subject. This is the interval scaling principle.

The rating scale is suitable for measuring preferences for both chronic and temporary health states. Chronic states should be described to the subject as permanent from age of onset until death, with the age of onset and death given. All chronic states with the same age of onset and death are then grouped together and measured relative to each other. Chronic states with different ages of onset and/or death can be measured by using several groups. Each group must have two additional chronic states as reference states for the scale added to it. These might be 'healthy (from age of onset until death' and 'death at age of onset'. The scale is then measured from 0 assigned to the worst health state of the group and 1 assigned to the best (see Figure 1). The subject is asked to select the best and worst health states from the group and then locate the other states on the scale relative to each other, according to the interval scaling principle described above.

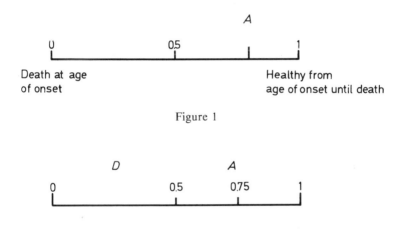

Figure 1

Figure 2

If death is considered the worst state of health and is placed at 0 on the scale, the preference value for each of the other states is simply the scale value associated with its placement. Suppose *A* represents a given chronic state, as shown in Figure 1, then the preference value can be read from the scale, which in this case is 0.8. However, it may be the case that death *D* is not considered the worst state and hence is repositioned as depicted in Figure 2 reflecting the subject who prefers to be dead than to be in certain specified chronic states. In this case the preference value for chronic state *A* must be recalculated so that a new position for *A* relative to *D* can be established on the scale. This may be obtained by applying the formula

$$\frac{X - D}{1 - D}$$

where X denotes the scale placement of the health state. This will give a measure of the ratio of the preference value to the new scale value. Thus, a preference value of 0.8 may, in this case, be translated into:

$$\frac{0.8 - 0.2}{1 - 0.2}$$

resulting in a placement value on the scale of 0.75 (Figure 2).

When preferences for temporary health states are measured on a rating scale, the states are described to the subject as being of a specified duration after which the person returns to normal health. All temporary health states of the same duration and with the same age of onset are grouped together and measured relative to each other. Temporary health states with different durations and/or ages of onset can be measured using multiple groups.

Each group requires the additional state 'healthy' to be added to it. The subject is asked to locate the best health state (which presumably would be healthy) at one end of the scale and the worst temporary health state at the other. The remaining temporary states are then located on the scale using the aforementioned interval scale principle.

This procedure is sufficient if the programmes being evaluated involve only morbidity and not mortality and in circumstances when it is not necessary to compare the findings with programmes that do involve mortality. If, however, this is not the case and mortality is encountered then the interval preference values for temporary states must be transformed on to the standard 0–1 health preference scale. To achieve this the worst temporary health state is redefined as a chronic state of the same duration and its preference value is measured by the method described for chronic states. Through the use of a positive linear transformation, that is, increment by a unit value of 1, the values for the remaining states can then be transformed on to the standard 0–1 health preference scale. (This procedure is akin to that of converting degrees Fahrenheit to degrees Centigrade.)

Standard Gamble

The 'Standard Gamble technique', based on the work of von Neumann and Morgenstern (1953) is used widely as a general measure for utilities and preferences. In recent years, it has been used in the field of health to measure preferences for different health states. Using this technique, subjects are asked to choose between a gamble, with a desirable outcome, with risk P, and a less desirable outcome, with risk $1-P$, and a certain option of intermediate desirability. The subject is asked what probability of getting the desirable or less desirable outcome will make him indifferent between the gamble and the certainty.

By way of illustration, subjects may be presented with the question:

Suppose you have a choice between living t years in health state A, or taking a gamble between a P-chance of t years in perfect health (H) and a $1-P$ chance of t years in state B (which might be coma or some other extreme reference state). What probability, P, would make you indifferent between the sure thing and the gamble?

The value of P corresponding to the best outcome, perfect health, is 1, and the value of P corresponding to the worst outcome, B, is 0. On answering the question the subject provides a number, P, that can be used as the weight assigned to health state A.

The 'standard gamble' technique can be used in the health field to measure preferences for both chronic and temporary health states. Figure 3 illustrates the method for measuring chronic states preferred to death. The subject faces two alternatives. Alternative one is a treatment with two possible outcomes: at a probability P the patient will return to normal health and live for an additional t years, or at a probability $(1-P)$ the patient will die immediately. Alternative two has the certain outcome of chronic state B for life (t years). Probability P is varied until the subject is indifferent between the two alternatives. At which point the preference value for chronic state B, (h_B), is simply P ($h_B = P$).

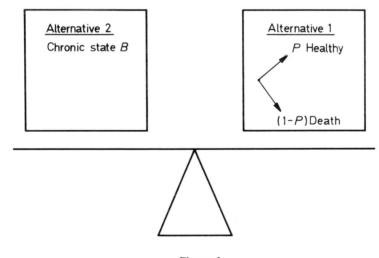

Figure 3

For measuring chronic states considered worse than death the standard gamble method must be slightly modified. This is illustrated in Figure 4. Here the

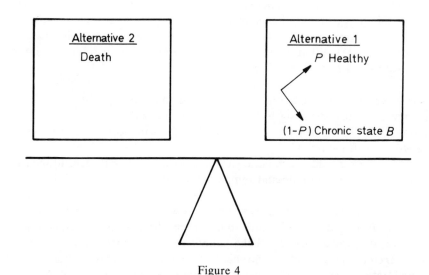

Figure 4

gamble alternative (alternative 1) leads to outcomes healthy, at probability P, or chronic state B at probability $(1-P)$. The certain alternative leads to death.

Torrance outlines one way in which this choice may be represented to the subject. Let the subject imagine he is faced with a rapidly progressing terminal disease, which if left untreated will quickly lead to death. A treatment is available, however, with the probability P of returning the patient to full health, and probability $(1-P)$ of leaving the subject irreversibly in chronic state B. As before, probability P is varied until the subject is indifferent between the uncertain and the certain alternatives. At this point the preference value for chronic state B is given by the formula:

$$\frac{h(D) \; - \; Ph(H)}{1 \; - \; P}$$

where $h(D)$ denotes the preference value for death and $h(H)$ the preference value for health.

Figure 5 illustrates the standard gamble approach to measuring preferences for temporary health states. As before, the subject faces two alternatives. Alternative 1 is a treatment with two possible outcomes: at probability P the patient returns to normal health, and at probability $(1 - P)$ the patient suffers from the worst temporary health state, K. Alternative 2 has the certain outcome of an intermediate temporary health state, J. The subject selects probability, P, at which point he is indifferent between the two alternatives. In this way the

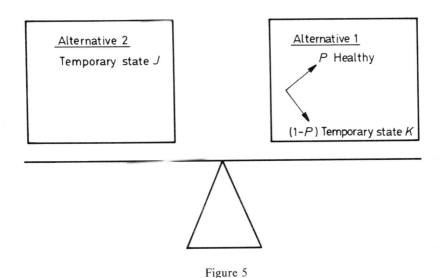

Figure 5

intermediate temporary health state (J) is measured relative to the best state (healthy) and the worst temporary health state (K).

Using the procedure outlined above, the preference value for temporary health state J is given by the formula

$$h_J = P - (1 - P)h_K$$

When mortality is not involved, h_K, the preference value for the worst temporary health state, can be set equal to 0 and hence the preference value for temporary health state J is simply $h_J = P$. However, when mortality is a consideration and it is desirable to relate these values to the 0–1 dead–healthy scale, state K must be redefined as a short duration chronic state, followed by death, and be measured on the 0–1 scale using the technique outlined for chronic states. This, in turn, provides a value for h_K which can then be used in the formula to enable the value h_J to be calculated.

Time Trade-off

The 'time trade-off' technique, pioneered by Torrance, is similar to the standard gamble technique in that it is based on paired comparison and allows the analyst to derive preference values implicitly, based on the subjects' responses to decision situations. It differs, however, in that no probabilities are involved.

The subject is presented with two alternatives and asked to select the most preferred. Alternative 1 offers the subject a particular outcome for a specified length of time followed by death, and alternative 2 offers a different outcome for a different length of time. The time is varied until the respondent is indifferent between the two alternatives.

As with the standard gamble and rating techniques, this approach can be used to measure preferences for both chronic and temporary health states. Figure 6 illustrates the application of the time trade-off technique for chronic states preferred to death. Alternative 1 is chronic state A for time t (i.e. the life expectancy of an individual with the chronic condition) followed by death, and alternative 2 is healthy for time X, where Xt, followed by death. Time X is varied until the subject is indifferent between the two alternatives at which point the preference value for chronic state A (hA), is given by

$$\frac{X}{t}$$

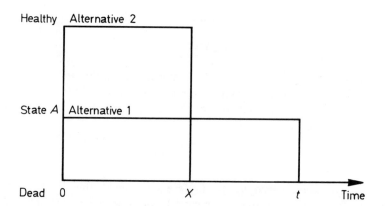

Figure 6

Figure 7 illustrates the procedure for the determination of preference values for chronic states preferred to death. Here the subject is asked to determine the time X such that he/she is indifferent between alternative 1, which represents healthy for time X (where Xt) followed by chronic state A until time t, followed by death, and alternative 2, which is to die immediately after birth. At the point of indifference the preference value for chronic state A (hA) is given by the formula:

$$\frac{X}{X - t}$$

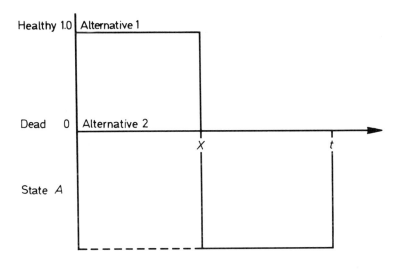

Figure 7

which is derived by equating the two alternatives,

$$1.0X + hA(t - X) = 0$$

and solving for hA.[*]

The application of the time trade-off technique to measure preferences for temporary health states is illustrated in Figure 8. The intermediate temporary health state (J) is measured relative to the best state (healthy) and the worst temporary health state (K). The subject has a choice of two alternatives: alternative 1 is intermediate temporary health state J for time t (the time duration specified for temporary states) followed by healthy, and alternative 2 is temporary state K for time X (where Xt) followed by healthy. The time X is varied until the respondent is indifferent between the two alternatives, at which point the preference value for temporary state J (h_1) is given by

$$\frac{1 - (1 - hK)X}{t}$$

---

[*] Torrance (1984) points out that in practice one difficulty encountered in this procedure is that although it imposes an upper limit of 1.0 on states preferred to death, it imposes no comparable lower limit on states dispreferred to death. One solution to this is to scale the preference values of those states considered worse than death, so that the worst possible state is assigned a preference value of -1.0.

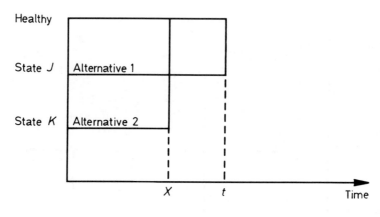

Figure 8

If $h_K = 0$, that is, the worst temporary health state is set equal to 0, h_J equals

$$\frac{1 - X}{t}$$

If the preference values for the temporary health states are to be transferred to the 0–1, dead–healthy scale, then the worst temporary health state must be redefined as a short duration chronic state and measured by the method previously described for chronic states.

As suggested, the rating scale, standard gamble and time trade-off techniques can all be applied to produce interval scales of utility. However, the measurement of utilities or preferences for health is clearly a complex and controversial task. Debate continues over the most appropriate use of those techniques considered here and some investigators have opted for alternative approaches. Of particular interest is a method used by Rosser and Kind (1978) in which subjects were asked to provide a ratio of undesirability of pairs of health states so as to produce a ratio scale of utility. A similar technique is the 'equivalence technique' whereby subjects are asked to identify their point of indifference between keeping alive a group of people in a 'standard state' of perfect health and a larger group, whose size is defined by the subject, of less well people.

Are the Utilities Valid?

The utility values or numerical weights assigned to different health states should, according to Torrance (1976) be non-arbitrary, community-based, scientifically measured values reflecting the relative desirability of various states of health. This requires the availability of a reliable and valid measurement instrument(s) which can be used on the general public to quantify the preferences for the relevant states of health.

With this in mind Torrance (1976) carried out an empirical investigation of three of the more commonly administered measurement techniques: he assessed the category method (an application of the rating scale) the standard gamble technique and the time trade-off technique for their feasibility, validity and comparability. Each health state selected for use in the study was described in a scenario outlining the physical, emotional and social characteristics of the state, and three groups acted as judges: a stratified sample of the population of Hamilton, Ontario; graduates from McMaster University; and patients involved in a local home dialysis programme.

The feasibility of each technique was determined by its acceptability to the judges, its ease of use for the interviewers and its cost. Taking the first of these criteria, the subjects' willingness to go through with the interview in all three cases, reflected their acceptability for use on the general public. However, there were noticeable differences in the ease with which the subjects found the techniques—the time trade-off technique proving to be the easiest, the standard gamble questions proving somewhat more difficult and the category scaling proving most difficult.

The professional interviewers found all three techniques easy to learn and straightforward to administer, although the use of a probability wheel was considered essential to enable the administration of the standard gamble technique. (A probability wheel is an adjustable disc with two sectors, each a different colour, constructed so that the relative size of the two sectors can be easily changed to reflect the relative probability of the alternative outcomes).

Turning to the cost encountered in the application of the three techniques, the standard gamble and time trade off approaches are inherently expensive, being both time-consuming and requiring an interview for administration. The category method, by comparison, is relatively cheap in that it is less time-consuming and has the potential for being used in the form of a mailed questionnaire.

Focusing on the reliability of the measurement techniques, if a utility can be measured more than once and produce identical results, the measurement technique is said to be reliable. In this study 'internal reliability' was tested by using replicated measurements[*] and 'test-retest reliability' was tested by retesting one group of subjects one year later.

When investigating 'internal reliability' the question arises of whether the change of the measurement is sufficient to disguise the replication from the

---

[*] This was not possible for the category scaling technique and hence there were no internal reliability measures for this method.

subject and yet at the same time insufficient so as not to affect the characteristic being measured. Since no subjects complained of questions being repeated the first objective appeared to be satisfied. However, statistical analysis of the difference between the original measurements and the replications indicated that in this study with the time trade-off technique 'the replicated measurement contained a content change such that the modified question was measuring a slightly different phenomenon'. Furthermore, it was suggested that, had the sample sizes for the standard gamble been larger, the same conclusion would probably have been achieved.

One year test-retest reliability gave a coefficient of 0.53 for the standard gamble, 0.62 for time trade-off and 0.49 for the category technique. Although the time trade-off technique can be seen to have the highest coefficient of test-retest reliability, the difference is not significant at the 0.05 confidence level. In Churchill's (1984) study, a 6-week test-retest correlation coefficient produced values ranging from 0.628 to 0.802. This might indicate that people's preferences shift over time.

Turning to validity, if the measurement technique actually measures what it claims to measure, in this case the utility or strength of a subject's preference for certain health states, it is said to be valid. 'Criterion validity', in which a new measure is assessed against a 'well-accepted' measure, was applied in this study with the standard gamble technique taken to represent the latter. The criterion validity of the time trade-off technique, as determined by the coefficient of validity (i.e. the product moment correlation coefficient between the measure under investigation and the criterion measure) was concluded to be 'satisfactory'. On the other hand, the criterion validity of the category method was found to be 'significantly poorer', and when recalculated using the time trade-off as the 'well-accepted' measure, the results were not significantly improved. This seems to suggest that at least for the category method, criterion validation is unsatisfactory.

Finally, the comparability of the three techniques was assessed in terms of whether or not they produce the same values, and if not whether the values derived are related in some systematic way so as to enable conversion curves to be constructed. When addressing this question to the measurement of population mean values, the time trade-off technique appeared to give equivalent results to the standard gamble technique, with a relationship between the two measures of standard gamble = time trade-off. However, when the question was addressed to the measurement of individual values the relationship was 'not so clear, but it seems likely that the same function may hold'.

The category scaling technique produced significantly different values for both individual and population mean values from those derived by either of the other two techniques. That said, however, there were systematic differences, for population mean values, between measures obtained by category scaling and those obtained by the time trade-off.

All this suggests that the time trade-off technique is the best of the three methods tested for measuring preferences for health states, with the standard gamble technique coming a close second. This study, and others like it, also serves a useful purpose in highlighting some of the inherent problems and uncertainties encountered in preference measurement. By way of example, differences in demographic characteristics such as age, sex, religion, etc., cannot fully account for the not insignificant differences in individual's health state preferences. Sackett and Torrance (1978) found a standard deviation between scores of about 0.30 for individual preferences among the public for a single health state. This not withstanding, the differences are less apparent among more homogenous subjects with a good knowledge of the health state. In application of the time trade-off technique (Torrance 1976, 1984) 29 home dialysis rating the home dialysis scenario resulted in a standard deviation of 0.18 compared to 0.28 for the general public.*

Applications and Discussion

The evaluation of health states by 'psychometric methods' is an exciting, innovative feature of current research on health indicators. As derived here, the values have the interval scale property which makes them useful for evaluative research and for projecting and comparing the benefits of alternative health programmes. It will doubtless be some time before measurement techniques have been developed which satisfy more fully criteria for reliability, validity, comparability and generalizability of social preferences (Patrick *et al.*, 1973) and the indices that they produce are accepted as valid inputs to decision-making. However, if further research is successful in developing health status indices which are acceptable to decision-makers, then clearly they will be powerful tools for all aspects of health care policy-making.

It was less than two decades ago when, in one of the earliest recorded applications, Klarman *et al.* (1968) introduced the concept of 'quality adjusted' life years gained in a cost effectiveness analysis of different treatments for renal failure. It was assumed that one year of life gained by transplant was equivalent to 1.25 years gained by dialysis, reflecting the higher quality of life under transplantation. Since then, there has been a rapid increase in the literature concerned with measuring the quality of life and research has progressed a long way.

Rosser (1983) provides a historical review of health indicators that claim to be direct assessments of a population's health. Under the heading, 'The Phase of Cardinal Measurement' the classic paper of Bush and his colleague (Fanshel and Bush, 1970) is discussed. They made a significant contribution

---

* This problem of differences between individual preferences can largely be overcome by taking the mean value of a large group of subjects.

using scaling techniques to develop a health index (formerly the Function Status Index and lately the Index of Wellbeing), which has since been modified and utilized in several applications including a tuberculosis prevention and treatment programme in New York (Fanshel and Bush, 1970), a phenylketonuria (PKU) screening programme (Bush *et al.*, 1973) and a large household survey (Kaplan *et al.*, 1976). Reynolds *et al.*, (1974) also claimed to have applied a modified version of the index in a survey of two counties in Alabama.

Card's group in Glasgow focused primarily on the measurement of utilities of states of illness for the purpose of formalizing clinical decisions, by way of incorporating the utility values into decision models. In particular they studied gastro-intestinal diseases and utilities of head injury; furthermore they antici-pated the conversion of utilities into money equivalents for use in CBA (Card, 1975) as did Culyer *et al.* in York (1971, 1972).

At about the same time as Bush began his prolific research, Torrance's group at McMaster University published a cost-utility model (Torrance *et al.*, 1972) which has since been further developed and applied to several health care pro-grammes including tuberculosis screening, haemolytic disease, Rhesus disease, renal dialysis and more recently neonatal intensive care of very-low-birth-weight infants. In addition two surveys of the general public to measure health state utilities have been carried out with one being based on a multi-attribute health state classification system (as previously described).

Further contributions in this field of work have been made by Rosser, Watts and Kind, who have focused particularly on indicators of hospital performance (Rosser and Watts, 1972; Rosser, 1976). They used two scaling methods, psy-chometric and behavioural. The former was based on magnitude estimation but included a lengthy interview procedure devised by Gibbs and Wishlade in their work on crime seriousness, and the latter, as already mentioned, was obtained by the analysis of legal awards for non-pecuniary consequences of personal in-jury and industrial accidents and disease. (This scaling method is significant in that unlike those described it reflects actual behaviour, and values inferred from an existing resource allocation process.) Thus research into health status measurement has made considerable progress in a relatively short space of time, and yet there are still a number of controversial and unresolved issues.

To begin with, the whole concept of combining the impact of a given health care activity on morbidity and mortality into a single measure (QALYs) gained is still debatable. It needs to be justified methodologically and ethically. It has to be established that the users of the studies fully understand the trade-offs built into the calculations. Secondly, in measuring utilities the question arises of whose values should count? That is, who should place values on states of health? To provide an answer to this question it must be established whether there are differences in opinion about the severity of illness between individuals and between different socio-economic groups and, if there are any differences, can they be aggregated or are they mutually exclusive? A third, and particularly important, issue concerns the specificity or generalizability of the utility values. Can a universal set of health state utilities be determined and used in all studies or does each study require its own utilities? Finally one must ask which technique is best to use and whether they are subject to different biases (such as risk aversion in the case of the standard gamble technique and time preference in the time trade-off technique).

The purpose of this chapter has been to expose some of the techniques currently being developed and utilized in the determination of health state utilities for use in economic appraisal. It has been demonstrated that health state preferences can be measured using these techniques, albeit somewhat imprecisely. However, as the impact of health care activities on the quality of life plays an increasingly important role, so the need to evaluate this objective becomes more and more apparent. Whereas the benefits of medicines introduced in the 1940s and 1960s were easy to measure, in terms of reducing hospital costs, deaths and sickness absence payments, as depicted in the introduction to the proceedings of the Office of Health Economics meeting on the measurement of social benefits of medicine, 'there is now an overwhelming need to *quantify* the benefits of the "quality of life" medicines, of the 1980s' (Teeling Smith, 1983). In the allocation of scarce resources available to society, it is irresponsible to omit from economic appraisal, quality of life and other intangible benefits (which receive high priority in the hierarchy of objectives of health care providers and consumers) simply because of difficulties in measurement and evaluation.

References

Acton, J. P. (1973). Evaluating public programs to save lives; the case of heart attacks. Research Report R/73/02. Santa Monica: Rand Corporation.

Boyle, M. H., Torrance, G. W., Sinclair, J. C. and Horwood, S. P. (1983). *New England Journal of Medicine*, **308**, 1330–7.

Bush, J. W., Chen, M. M. and Patrick, D. L. (1973). Health Status Index in cost effectiveness: analysis of PKU programme. In *Health Status Indexes, Proceedings of a Conference conducted by Health Services Research.* (ed.) Berg, R. L.

Card, W. I. (1975). Ciba Foundation Symposium 34 (New Series), Amsterdam: Elsevier-Excerpta Medica.

Churchill, D. N., Morgan, J. and Torrance, G. W. (1984). *Peritoneal Dialysis Bulletin*, 20-23, January–March.

Culyer, A. J. (1978). *Measuring Health: Lessons for Ontario*, University of Toronto Press.

Culyer, A. J., Lavers, R. J. and Williams, A. (1971). *Social Trends*, **1**, 31–42, HMSO.

Culyer, A. J., Lavers, R. J. and Williams, A. (1972). Health Indicators. In *Social Indicators and Social Policy.* (ed.) Shonfield, A. and Shaw, S. London: Heinemann.

Drummond, M. (1984). Economic evaluation in the developement and promotion of medicines. Paper for Conference, New Challenge in Drugs Developement, Promotion and Innovation Strategies, held in Paris.

Fanshel, S. and Bush, J. W. (1970). A health status index and its application to health services outcomes. *Operations Research*, **18**, 1021–66.

Gibbs, R. J. (1972). Home Office Police Planning Organisation Report. No. 10/72, London: HMSO.

Grogono, A. W. and Woodgate, D. J. (1971). Index for measuring health, *Lancet*, 1024–26.

Harris, A. L., Cox, E. and Smith, R. W. (1971). *Handicapped and Impaired in Great Britain*, London: HMSO.

Kaplan, R. M. and Bush, J. W. (1982). *Health Psychology*, **1**, 61–80.

Kaplan, R. M., Bush, J. W. and Berry, C. C. (1976). *Health Services Research*, **11**, 478–507.

Karnofsky, D. A. and Burchenal, J. H. (1949). The clinical evaluation of chemotherapeutic agents in cancer. In *Evaluation of Chemotherapeutic Agents*. (ed.) Maclead, C. M., Columbia University Press.

Klarman, H. E., Francis, J. O's. and Rosenthal, G. D. (1968). *Medical Care*, **6**, 48–54.

Llewellyn-Thomas, M., Sutherland, H. J., Tibshirani, R., Ciampi, A., Till, J. E. and Boyd, N. F. (1982). *Medical Decision Making*, **2**, 449–62.

McNeil, B. J., Weichselbaum, R. and Pauker, S. G. (1981). *New England Journal of Medicine*, **305**, 982–7.

Mishan, E. (1971). *Journal of Political Economy*, **79**, 687–705.

Neumann, J. von and Morgenstern, D. (1953). *Theory of Games and Economic Behaviour*, 3rd edn. New York: Wiley.

Patrick, D. L., Bush, J. W. and Chen, M. M. (1973). Methods for measuring levels of well-being for a health status index. *Health Services Research*, **8**, 228–45.

Pliskin, J. S., Shepherd, D. S. and Weinstein, M. C. (1980). *Operations Research*, **28**, 206–24.

Reynolds, W. J., Rushing, W. A. and Miles, D. L. (1974). *Journal of Health and Social Behaviour*, **15**, 271–89.

Rosser, R. M. (1976). *Medical Care*, **14**, Supplement, 138–47.

Rosser, R. (1983). Issues of measurement in the design of health indicators: a review. In *Health Indicators* (ed.) Culyer, A. J. and Martin Robertson.

Rosser, R. and Watts, V. C. (1972). The measurement of hospital output. *International Journal of Epidemiology*, **1**, 361–8.

Rosser, R. M. and Kind, P. (1978). A scale evaluation of states of illness: is there a social consensus? *International Journal of Epidemiology*, **7**, 347–58.

Sackett, D. L. and Torrance, G. W. (1978). The utility of different health states as perceived by the general public. *Journal of Chronic Diseases*, **31**, 697–704.

Schelling, T. C. (1968). The life you save may be your own. In *Problems in Public Expenditure Analysis* (ed.) Samuel, B., Washington DC.

Spitzer, W. O., Dobson, J. J., Hall, J., Chesterman, E., Levy, J., Shepherd, R. and Battista, R. (1981). Measuring the quality of life of cancer patients. *Journal of Chronic Diseases*, **34**, 585–97.

Sutherland, H. J., Dunn, V. and Boyd, N. F. (1983). *Medical Decision Making*, **3**, 477–87.

Teeling Smith, G. (1983). *Measuring the Social Benefits of Medicine*, London: OHE.

Thaler, R. and Rosen, S. (1975). The value of saving a life: evidence from the labour market. In *Household Production and Consumption*, (ed.) Terleckyj, N., National Bureau of Economic Research.

Torrance, G. W. (1976). Social preferences for health states: an empirical evaluation of three measurement techniques. *Socio-Economic Planning Sciences*, **10**, 129–36.

Torrance, G. W. (1984). Health Status Measurement for economic appraisal. Paper presented to Health Economists' Study Group meeting, Aberdeen.

Torrance, G. W. and Zipursky, A. (In press) Clinics in perinatalogy.

Torrance, G. W., Thomas, W. H. and Sackett, D. L. (1972). *Health Services Research*, **7**, 118–133.

Torrance, G. W., Sackett, D. L. and Thomas, H. T. (1973). Utility maximisation model for program evaluation: a demonstration application. In *Health Status Indexes*, Proceedings of a Conference conducted by Health Services Research, (ed.) Berg, R. L.

Torrance, G. W., Boyle, M. H. and Horwood, S. P. (1982). *Operations Research*, **30**, 1043–69.

Wolfson, A. D., Sinclair, A. J., Bombardier, C. and McGeer, A. (1982). Preference measurement for functional status in stroke patients: inter-rater and inter-technique comparisons. In *Values and Long Term Care*, (eds.) Kane, R. and Kane, R., Washington DC: Health Publishers.

Measuring Health: A Practical Approach
Edited by G. Teeling Smith
© 1988 John Wiley & Sons Ltd

5

The Time Trade-off Approach to Health State Valuation

Martin Buxton and Joy Ashby
Health Economics Research Group, Brunel University, Uxbridge

Introduction

The process of measuring health involves at least two distinct elements—description of health states and their valuation. Both are the subject of much current research, in an international attempt to develop appropriate techniques. As yet no definitive approaches have emerged. Rather, there are a number of more or less well-proven methodologies and guidelines emerging.

This paper focuses on one main technique for valuation—the time trade-off, or TTO. It explains the technique, its development mainly in Canada, and a recent application in the UK. While primarily focused on TTO as a method of valuation it throws some comparative light on alternative valuation systems, and in discussing the divergent results emphasizes the interrelationship of valuation and the underlying description of health states. The technique is not claimed as a panacea for the problems of valuation but as an important weapon in the armoury to be targeted on the inevitably difficult problem of valuing health states.

The Time Trade-off Technique

In essence the time trade-off technique (TTO) approach is an equivalence technique which involves the subjects judging how many years in a state of full health are equivalent to a given number of years in a described imperfect state.

The procedure is at its simplest for chronic states considered better than death. Thus as in Figure 1:

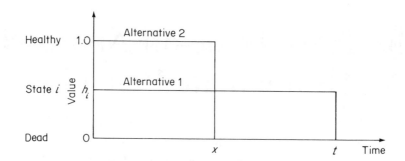

Figure 1. Time trade-off for a chronic health state preferred to death

The subject is offered two alternatives—alternative 1: state i for time t (life expectancy for an individual with the chronic condition) followed by death; and alternative 2: healthy for time $x < t$ followed by death. Time x is varied until the respondent is indifferent between the two alternatives, at which point the required preference value for state i is given by $h_i = x/t$. (Torrance , 1986, p.23)

Experimentally, in an interview, this point of indifference is usually recorded as lying midway between the closest pair of values between which preference for the alternative changes.

The technique can be adapted to accommodate states considered worse than death by finding the point of indifference between alternative 1: a variable period of healthy life followed by the poor health state followed by death and alternative 2: immediate death. In other words, how many years of healthy life are valued as compensating for the health state worse than death. Similarly, preferences for temporary health states can be measured relative to each other and then one of these treated as a short-term chronic state and measured relative to healthy and dead as outlined above.

While the TTO process is implicit (unlike, for example, the explicitness of a rating scale) the values are derived very simply from a response to decision situations requiring indication simply of preference (or absence of preference). Furthermore, the trade-off is not unlike the real choice sometimes offered by alternative therapies for a particular condition. For example, McNeil *et al.* (1981) used the TTO approach to illuminate the nature of the trade-offs involved in choosing between laryngectomy and radiation therapy for stage 3 carcinoma of the larynx. The former offers better survival but at a reduced quality of life (the loss of normal speech) while the latter offers poorer survival but with near normal quality of life.

One of its main attractions is that the TTO approach has been found in practice to be a very acceptable method of obtaining valuations. Torrance (1976) presents the results of a study comparing the use of three techniques for valuation: TTO, category scaling and the standard gamble. The TTO was as described above; the category scaling involved marking a line or linear analogue scale; the standard gamble, the widely used process first proposed by Neumann and Morgenstern (1953), offers paired choices involving a gamble of the certainty of imperfect health states versus the gamble of full health and death according to variable probabilities which are again adjusted to the point of indifference. Torrance concluded that the TTO method was the most acceptable of the three to the general public interviewed, who found it the easiest to answer. Measures of its reliability and validity were similar to that of the standard gamble which had been viewed as the accepted criterion for measurement of preferences. Overall he judged the TTO method as 'the best of the three tested for use on the general public in the measurement of social preferences for health states' (Torrance, 1976, p.135).

North American Development of the Technique

TTO and Scenarios

The first major use of the technique was in a study by Sackett and Torrance (1978). In this study ten different scenarios were valued, and each was considered as applying to one (or more) of three time durations. The interviews were conducted on a sample of 246 of the local general population in Hamilton, Ontario, using a stratified sampling frame. The main results are summarized in Table 1. (NB Not all scenarios were valued by all subjects.) In analysing the results Sackett and Torrance note a number of statistically significant differences between age and socio-economic groups. More importantly the results show that the utility of health state is statistically significantly time dependent and decreases as the length of time in the health state is extended. They also indicate statistically significant disease-labelling effects: 'tuberculosis' was preferred to an 'unnamed contagious disease' despite an otherwise identical health state scenario, while similarly 'mastectomy for injury' was preferred to 'mastectomy for breast cancer'. In addition the values of 34 dialysis patients were obtained: for all the dialysis scenarios the utilities derived from these patients who had experience of dialysis were higher than for the general population sample, and generally these differences were statistically significant.

Table 1. TTO health state utilities from Sackett and Torrance

Health state scenarios	Duration		
	3 Months	8 Years	Life
Depression	0.44	—	—
Home confinement for tuberculosis	0.68	—	—
Home confinement for unnamed contagious disease	0.65	—	—
Hospital confinement for tuberculosis	0.60	—	—
Hospital dialysis	0.62	0.56	0.32
Hospital confinement for unnamed contagious disease	0.56	0.33	0.16
Home dialysis	—	0.65	0.40
Kidney transplant	—	0.58	—
Mastectomy for breast cancer	—	0.48	—
Mastectomy for injury	—	0.63	—

Source: Sackett and Torrance, (1978), Table 2.

Since then the TTO technique has been used to value specific health state utilities for incorporation into economic evaluations of diverse interventions. For example, work on health states in treatments for end-stage renal disease (Churchill *et al.*, 1984); quality of life in cancer therapy (O'Connor *et al.*, 1985); and measurement of the quality of life impact on carers whose relatives received institutional respite care (Mohide *et al.*, 1987).

The use of scenarios as the basis of description has both advantages and disadvantages. The special characteristics of very diverse 'health' states can be reflected in the scenario description and the health state does not have to be forced into a predetermined and inevitably restrictive matrix of descriptors. There is therefore less danger of omitting factors important to the utility attached to particular health states. Thus it is easier to encompass in comparable utility valuations very different health state situations. If, and as appropriate, non-health-specific factors can be introduced into the scenario—age of subject, family responsibilities, etc.

However, there is a converse to this freedom. Evidence from a number of studies has shown the exact wording of the descriptions, the amount of detail provided, and the framing of the questions may influence the utilities obtained (e.g. Llewellyn-Thomas *et al.*, 1984). It would be wrong to suggest that a 'correct' method exists, but given the uncertainties Torrance suggests that:

the best current advice in measuring utilities on the general public is probably to use abbreviated descriptions to avoid cognitive overload, to supplement these with prior more detailed descriptions of the key phrases used in the abbreviated scenarios, and to avoid the framing bias by wording questions in a balanced (positive and negative) manner. (Drummond *et al.*, 1987, p.116)

Certainly it must be stressed that by focusing on the issue of valuation, TTO does not remove the problem of description.

TTO and a Multi-attribute Classification

However, TTO is not inherently linked to broad flexible scenarios. Other work has involved the development of a multi-attribute health classification and then the mapping of that classification into a single utility scale. Boyle *et al.*(1982) developed a system to classify and follow for life the outcomes of infants in an evaluation of neonatal intensive care. They produced a classification based on four attributes: physical function, role function, social-emotional function and health problems (see Figure 2). Each attribute has a number of levels so that each person can be classified at any point in time into one level on each attribute. With the attributes having 6, 5, 4 and 8 levels respectively, 960 possible health states exist. This represented too many 'scenarios' to value using holistic methods.

Instead multi-attribute utility (MAU) theory was used to derive values for each state from data on utilities attached to seven representative multi-attribute health states. These utilities had been elicited using the TTO technique on a sample of healthy adults in the community: (87 subjects provided the data used). From this a multiplicative function has been derived which enables the utility of any particular health state to be calculated according to the formula:

$$U = 1.42(m_1 \ m_2 \ m_3 \ m_4) - 0.42$$

using the multiplicative utility factors for the appropriate level of each attribute as set out in Table 2.

The advantage of the MAU system described above is that it appears to provide a relatively sensitive (960 combination) classification system with values attached, so that utility measurement need not necessarily be carried out for each new scenario involved in an empirical study. It provides, like the 'Rosser' matrix, off-the-peg utility valuations. Unlike the work of Rosser, the underpinning valuation process is that of the TTO.

The state of art of the MAU approach has been nicely summarized thus:

the formula given here is based on our best data and knowledge to date, but undoubtedly is not the last word. It can be very helpful as a simple and quick approximation, particularly when coupled with sensitivity analysis. (Drummond *et al.*, 1987, p.121)

X_1 Physical function: mobility and physical activity[a]

Level x_1	Code	Description
1	P1	Being able to get around the house, yard, neighbourhood or community WITHOUT HELP from another person; AND having NO limitation in physical ability to lift, walk, run, jump or bend
2	P2	Being able to get around the house, yard, neighbourhood or community WITHOUT HELP from another person; AND having SOME limitation in physical ability to lift, walk, run, jump or bend
3	P4	Being able to get around the house, yard, neighbourhood or community WITHOUT HELP from another person; AND NEEDING mechanical aids to walk or get around
4	P4	NEEDING HELP from another person in order to get around the house, yard, neighbourhood or community; AND having SOME limitations in physical ability to lift, walk, run, jump or bend
5	P5	NEEDING HELP from another person in order to get around the house, yard, neighbourhood or community; AND NEEDING mechanical aids to walk or get around
6	P6	NEEDING HELP from another person in order to get around the house, yard, neighbourhood or community; AND NOT being able to use or control the arms and legs

X_2 Role function: self-care and role activity[a]

Level x_2	Code	Description
1	R1	Being able to eat, dress, bathe, and go to the toilet WITHOUT HELP; AND having NO limitations when playing, going to school, working or in other activities
2	R2	Being able to eat, dress, bathe, and go to the toilet WITHOUT HELP; AND having SOME limitations when playing, going to school, working or in other activities
3	R3	Being able to eat, dress, bathe, and go to the toilet WITHOUT HELP; AND NOT being able to play, go to school or work
4	R4	NEEDING HELP to eat, dress, bathe, and go to the toilet AND having SOME limitations when playing, going to school, working or in other activities
5	R5	NEEDING HELP to eat, dress, bathe, and go to the toilet AND NOT being able to play, attend school or work

X_3 Social-emotional function: emotional wellbeing and social activity

Level x_3	Code	Description
1	S1	Being happy and relaxed most or all of the time, AND having an average number of friends and contacts with others
2	S2	Being happy and relaxed most or all of the time, AND having very few friends and little contact with others
3	S3	Being anxious or depressed some or a good bit of the time, AND having an average number of friends and contacts with others
4	S4	Being anxious or depressed some or a good bit of the time, AND having very few friends and contact with others

X_4 Health problem[b]

Level x_4	Code	Description
1	H4	Having no health problem
2	H2	Having a minor physical deformity or disfigurement such as scars on the face
3	H3	Needing a hearing aid
4	H4	Having a medical problem which causes pain or discomfort for a few days in a row every two months
5	H5	Needing to go to a special school because of trouble learning or remembering things
6	H6	Having trouble seeing even when wearing glasses
7	H7	Having trouble being understood by others
8	H8	Being blind OR deaf OR not able to speak

[a] Multiple choices within each description are applied to individuals as appropriate for their age. For example, a 3-year-old child is not expected to be able to get around the community without help from another person.

[b] Individuals with more than one health problem are classified according to the problem they consider the most serious.

Source: Drummond et al. (1987), Table 6.1.

Figure 2.   Multi-attribute utility health state classification

Table 2. MAU classification; multiplicative utility factors

Physical function		Role function		Social-emotional function		Health problem	
Level	Multiplicative utility factor m_1	Level	Multiplicative utility factor m_2	Level	Multiplicative utility factor m_3	Level	Multiplicative utility factor m_4
$P1$	1.00	$R1$	1.00	$S1$	1.00	$H1$	1.00
$P2$	0.91	$R2$	0.94	$S2$	0.96	$H2$	0.92
$P3$	0.81	$R3$	0.77	$S3$	0.86	$H3$	0.91
$P4$	0.80	$R4$	0.75	$S4$	0.77	$H4$	0.91
$P5$	0.61	$R5$	0.50			$H5$	0.86
$P6$	0.52					$H6$	0.84
						$H7$	0.83
						$H8$	0.74

Source: Drummond, Stoddart and Torrance, 1987, Table 6.2

A UK Application of the TTO

Background

There has been much interest recently in the UK in the use of QALYs as a conceptual device to assist decision-making. The advocacy of the criterion of 'cost per QALY' for prioritizing health care interventions within a fixed budget system has been forceful but controversial. Some of the opposition has been to the conceptual principle—but the argument for that principle is presented elsewhere in this volume (Chapter 11). Some opposition has focused on the appropriateness of the quality adjustment values (or health state utilities). Until recently, all the UK discussion of QALYs has been based on the 'Rosser' matrix of values obtained by psychometric scaling techniques of magnitude estimation from a group of 70 subjects (see Kind *et al.*, 1982 and Chapter 3).

The Health Economics Research Group (HERG) at Brunel University decided that it was important to test empirically in the UK alternative methods of obtaining valuations, and to explore the effects of different methods on the values obtained, and the way values might vary systematically between different groups. Given the extensive Canadian experience of the TTO, the preference for this approach indicated by a number of the North American studies, and the fact that TTO valuations of health states were incorporated into 'cost per QALY' league tables as an aid to decision-making there, it seemed strange that the TTO approach had been so ignored in the UK. HERG therefore set up a small initial study. It had two main purposes—the first methodological, the second a substantive input into on-going evaluation work. These were:

(a) to explore the time trade-off technique in a UK context with UK subjects, and to compare its conceptual validity, practical implementation and substantive results with those that might be obtained from the use of the Rosser psychometric valuations;

(b) to obtain quality adjustment values for breast cancer patients by surveying and synthesizing existing qualitative information from various trials and studies of breast cancer patients, as a basis for describing the relevant health states; applying the time trade-off method with various individuals (forming representation samples) to elicit their relative valuations of these health states of breast cancer patients; comparing the values so obtained with the results from applying the same information to existing Rosser psychometric valuation matrices.

Construction of the Scenarios

A literature survey on quality of life of breast cancer patients after treatment indicated a large number of studies that had relevant but rather limited material on quality of life. Some of the studies gave evidence of relatively short-term or transient effects of the treatments (surgery, radiotherapy and chemotherapy). We chose to focus on the more important long-term effects of diagnosis and treatment, and focused on evidence relating to a period approximately one year after treatment on the basis that this would be indicative of the long-term health states. Particular use was made of the evidence from seven studies: Craig *et al.* (1974); Winick and Robbins (1977); Morris *et al.* (1977); Maguire *et al.* (1978); Greer *et al.* (1979); van Dam *et al.* (1980); and Meyerowitz *et al.* (1983).

On the basis of these, a number of scenarios were constructed reflecting a range of possible surgical treatments and outcomes. The format adopted was built on the experience of Torrance and his colleagues. The scenarios reflected the physical, emotional and social health states of typical breast cancer patients. After discussion with various clinicians and others with direct experience of such patients, five scenarios were agreed plus a baseline healthy scenario. Appendix A sets out two of the scenarios in full by way of illustration and Figure 3 presents a summary of the way the scenarios were differentiated.

The Interview

A detailed interview schedule was developed incorporating the time trade-off exercise in which the scenarios were handled as chronic health states preferred to death. The interview incorporated two main elements following Torrance and Mohide (1985). The first required the subjects to read and rank order the scenarios. The second stage was to obtain the TTO values for each of the five scenarios (taking them in the rank order, that the subject had previously indicated, from best situation to worst). To assist the subject the interviewer

	W 'Williams'	L 'Lewis'	P 'Powell'	K 'King'	T 'Thomas'
Surgery:	Lumpectomy	Simple mastectomy with recon- struction	Simple mastectomy	Lumpectomy	Simple mastectomy
Physical restriction:	None	None	None	Limited arm movement	Limited arm movement
Psychological reaction:	Good	Good	Fairly good	Very poor	Very poor
Social effects:	None	None	Slight	Severe	Severe

Figure 3.   Summary structure of breast cancer scenarios

had a visual aid which displayed sliding scales of lengths of life alongside the relevant scenarios. The future years of life for the scenarios were based on the average life expectancy of the women in the subject's own age-range, and the scales on the visual aid were determined accordingly. The subject was first asked for his/her preference between 20, 30, 40 or 50 years (depending upon the subject's age) of full health situation as compared with the same number of years of the first 'post-cancer' description. Assuming preference for the full health state, the choice was then changed to the other end of the scale of 2 (3/4/5) years of perfect health as compared to the 20 (30/40/50) of the 'post-cancer' health state. The interview then 'ping-ponged' back and forth between high (but decreasing) and low (but increasing) lengths of good-quality life as compared to the fixed length of the 'poorer' health state, until the points were established between which a switch of preference occurred. This process was then repeated for the other four scenarios, in each case compared to full health.

With basic socio-economic questions at the beginning of the interview, and 'sweep-up' questions on their previous experience of breast cancer or breast cancer patients and their reactions to the exercise, the interview generally lasted 20–25 minutes.

Choice of Subjects: Whose Values?

In this particular application with its focus on methodology, the choice of subjects reflected two considerations. The first was a desire to be able to compare results broadly with those of other health state valuation studies particularly the work of Rosser and her colleagues. The second was the pragmatic factor of ease of access within a low-budget study. Through the local general hospital access was obtained to groups of nurses, hospital doctors and general practitioners. In addition a sample of the total university workforce was invited to be interviewed as a proxy for a general population with no professional experience of the effects of the treatments. Table 3 shows the groups and numbers interviewed by age and sex. All were asked whether they would be prepared to be reinterviewed after a period of weeks; all but one agreed and a sample of 35 were reinterviewed. (Reinterviews are indicated in parentheses in the table.)

Table 3. Characteristics of subjects

| | Subject groupings | | | | |
	Nurses	Hospital doctors	General practitioners	University staff	Total
Males					
<25	—	2	—	—	2
25–34	—	5	2	—	7
35–44	1	—	6 (1)	5 (4)	12 (5)
45–54	—	—	2 (1)	2 (1)	4 (2)
55–64	—	1 (1)	6 (2)	3 (2)	10 (5)
Total	1	8	26 (4)	10 (7)	35 (12)
Females					
<25	6	—	—	—	6
25–34	11 (1)	4 (1)	2 (1)	—	17 (3)
35–44	15 (5)	5 (2)	4	—	24 (7)
45–54	12 (3)	2 (1)	2	16 (7)	32 (11)
55–64	4 (1)	1	—	2 (1)	7 (2)
Total	48 (10)	12 (4)	8 (1)	18 (8)	86 (23)
Total	49 (10)	20 (5)	24 (5)	28 (15)	121 (35)

(Retest interviews in brackets)

In applying utility values, there is a value judgement to be made as to whose values should count. If the choices involved are for the care of an individual patient then presumably his/her values should be used, or values most likely to be a close representation of them. In making planning choices for the care of groups, then the most appropriate value base is less obvious. A political choice has to be made as to whether the appropriate values are those of the groups directly affected, society at large or the decision-makers who are responsible for the service. It is an important conceptual problem, but until we have a better understanding of how, or if, values differ between groups, we know neither the practical importance nor the consequences of the choice of values.

The Results

The results of this study have been formally presented in Buxton *et al.*, 1987, and it is to that source the readers are directed for a full statistical analysis. Table 4 summarizes the results. In this report, the focus is on the general implications for the TTO approach, what the study suggests about the nature

Table 4. Rank orderings and values: all subjects ($n = 121$)

Patient scenarios	Rank ordering (percentages)					TTO values		
	1	2	3	4	5	Mean	95% confidence interval	Median
W	67.8	23.1	8.3	0.8	—	0.722	0.669–0.775	0.850
L	23.1	62.9	14.0	—	—	0.695	0.640–0.750	0.850
P	5.0	19.0	74.4	1.7	—	0.680	0.623–0.737	0.850
K	—	0.8	1.7	77.8	19.8	0.271	0.212–0.330	0.150
T	—	—	1.7	19.1	79.3	0.237	0.182–0.292	0.050

1 = most desirable health state
5 = least desirable health state

Statistical significance of difference in mean values:
(P values from t test for difference between means)

	L	P	K	T
W	0.24	0.05	0.00	0.00
L		0.32	0.00	0.00
P			0.00	0.00
L				0.03

and variability of values and the relationship of these results to other reported health state values.

The initial rank ordering exercise indicates at one and the same time a large degree of overall agreement in preference ordering, combined with a wide range of individual subject variation. Figure 4 presents graphically the rank ordering of the scenarios. While for each scenario there was at least 60 per cent of the subjects who agreed on its rank position, there was recorded divergence from these orderings with, for example, individual subjects appearing to judge the 'Williams' scenario not just as the commonly agreed first rank, but also second, third and indeed fourth. A number of possible explanations may exist for the outliers. They may reflect a failure to understand the ranking exercise— although the chances of that are minimized by the interview instructions. They may reflect a failure to absorb the full characteristics of the scenarios and hence a judgement based only on part of the information—'cognitive overload'. Or, they may simply and accurately reflect unconventional values. In looking at the TTO values for a particular scenario (as in Figure 5) there is again evidence of a wide range of individual valuations alongside a clear central tendency. The nature of the distribution does emphasize that in focusing on any single value to represent the observed range a wealth of detail is inevitably lost, and that within constrained ranges of values the choice of measure of central tendency is important. Figure 6 shows the means and their 95 per cent confidence limits, and medians for the value of each scenario, and emphasizes the difference between mean and median values.

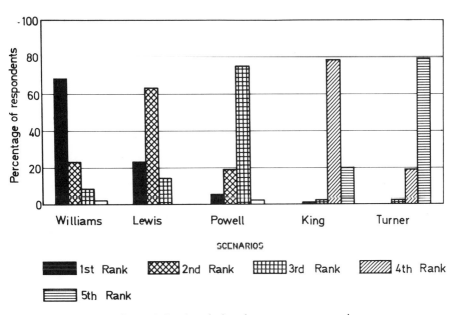

Figure 4. Rank ordering: breast cancer scenarios

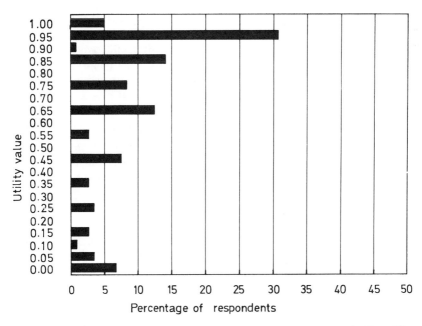

Figure 5. Frequency distribution of values: breast cancer scenario 'Powell'

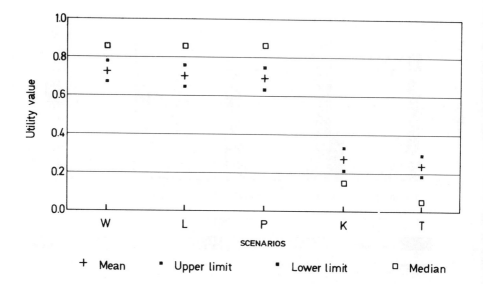

Figure 6.   Utility values: breast cancer scenarios means, 95 per cent confidence limits, and medians

The Canadian TTO literature normally presents means; the Rosser matrix is based on median values. While the choice is often argued on a technical basis, it is not simply a technical matter. Use of the median effectively gives an equal weight to each subject's assessment of the utility. The mean is influenced by strength of individual preference (or magnitude of value). A modal value would reflect the most commonly accepted value. The choice between these is in effect a further value judgement of the researcher.

Analysing the results on a disaggregated basis by professional group, age or sex produced few statistically significant differences. While by no means definitive, the results lend further support to the impression from previous studies that there are no large systematic differences in values between groups.

Comparison with other Values

In terms of tests of reliability and validity (see Buxton *et al.*, 1987) this UK study seemed to have produced results on a par with earlier work of Torrance. Here, as in previous studies, test-retest values are not as good as might be hoped for. But again there is more than one possible explanation of this. It may reflect inaccuracy in valuation resulting from the TTO methodology, or it may represent substantive change in values over time. In that the interview with its ranking and TTO processes may be the first time that the individuals have consciously considered their values and preferences in this matter, it would not be surprising if the process itself may lead to some change in perceived values, and perhaps further retesting might show a stabilization of values. (This incidentally is a problem that applies to any method for eliciting information on values.)

In terms of previous values for similar scenarios as shown in Table 1, Sackett and Torrance looked at long-term valuations for mastectomy for breast cancer, and obtained a value of 0.48 (based on an eight-year duration). This is just about midway between the mean values in this study for the most comparable scenarios of Powell and Turner (0.68 and 0.24).

As a comparison with alternative approaches to valuation, the scenarios were rated independently by six researchers from the University of York to place them in a cell of the Rosser matrix and by eleven researchers from McMaster University to assess them in terms of the multi-attribute utility classification described above. In each case, there was a high degree of agreement as to which was the appropriate classification for the scenarios, although there was some difficulty in appropriately placing the scenarios on the health problem attribute of the MAU classification. The resulting values (compared with the TTO means and medians) are shown in Figure 7.

This suggests a fairly close accordance between the TTO-median values and the MAU values for scenarios W, L and P but not so for K and T. For these the MAU values are a little closer to the TTO-mean values. There is no accordance with the Rosser values—and for K and T the TTO values appear quite at odds with the Rosser values.

Various hypotheses have been posed as possible explanations of all, or part, of the considerable differences between the values for the scenarios derived from our TTO work and from the use of the Rosser matrix, and to a lesser extent the MAU values. These include:

(a) the effect of 'labelling' the disease—values may be lowered by describing the health state as being due to cancer (see Sackett and Torrance, 1978): neither of the other sets of valuations would include a 'labelling' effect;
(b) the current Rosser valuations and to a lesser extent the MAU values may not adequately allow for psychological distress that is evident in scenarios K and T;
(c) the TTO values are being 'contaminated' by respondents 'disbelieving' the hypothetical lengths of life quoted and substituting their own expectations of actual prognosis;
(d) a high discount rate for the value of future years of life is being implicitly incorporated into the TTO comparison: this factor would also be at work in the TTO-based MAU valuations;
(e) the scalings may be logarithmically related, reflecting a prothetic relationship between the scales, possibly implying that the TTO-based values be on a scale with the characteristics of an interval scale rather than a true ratio scale (see Patrick *et al.*, 1973).

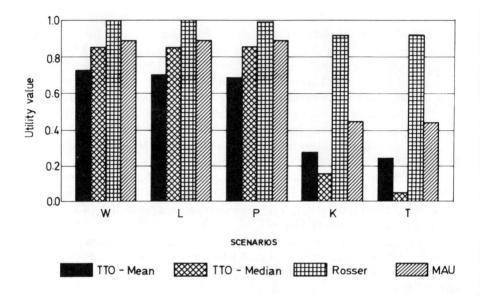

Figure 7. Utility values: breast cancer scenarios mean and median TTO, Rosser and MAU

Each of these hypotheses warrants further investigation and some of this is underway as part of the next phase of the research, involving interviews which include a 'debriefing' as to the factors that influenced subjects' responses.

As an exploratory test of the hypothesis about scaling, a logarithmic transformation of the Rosser values was made (see Buxton *et al.*, 1987, Table 10 for mathematical details). Figure 8 shows that in fact the MAU values and the log-transformed Rosser values are quite close. This lends support to the hypothesis that there is a scaling effect with a logarithmic relationship between the two scales, and possibly by extension between TTO and magnitude estimation scaling in general.

Such a relationship may be important, not because at the moment it is easy to say that one or other scale is thus correct in its original form, but as evidence that there are systematic and explicable relationships emerging between the value sets. The values being obtained in such independent, methodologically varying studies, though numerically quite different, may be logically and statistically related. The values are not arbitrary or random as some critics might wish to suggest.

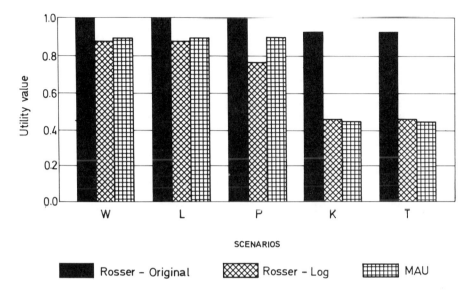

Figure 8. Utility values: breast cancer scenarios Rosser, log-transformed Rosser, and MAU

Conclusions

At this stage, it would be a bold person who argued that any researcher has a definitive, generally applicable set of values. But methodologies exist for obtaining values, for exploring differences, and beginning to understand the factors that influence health state valuation. It would be surprising if the measurement of individual values of complex health states was easy, if there were not considerable differences between individuals, and if the process of elicitation did not influence the values obtained. But such difficulties are no reason to remain in ignorance.

On the basis of the work carried out so far in the Health Economics Research Group at Brunel University we believe that there is much to be gained from building on the Canadian experience with the TTO approach. TTO provides a relatively easy and acceptable technique for eliciting values; its relative ease of use opens up on the one hand the possibility of large-scale sampling to explore differences in values and on the other smaller scale testing of the detailed effects of the form, content and context of scenarios. Both are urgently needed if health state values are to be routinely incorporated into policy analysis.

References

Boyle, M.H., Torrance, G.W., Sinclair, J.C. *et al.* (1982). Economic evaluation of neonatal intensive care of very low birth-weight infants. *New England Journal of Medicine*, **308**(22), 1330–1337.

Buxton, M.J., Ashby, J. and O'Hanlon, M.(1987). *Alternative Methods of Valuing Health States: A Comparative Analysis Based on an Empirical Study Using the Time Trade-off Approach in Relation to Health States One Year After Treatment for Breast Cancer.* Paper presented to the Third Annual Meeting of the International Society of Technology Assessment in Health Care, Rotterdam, 21–22 May 1987, HERG, Brunel University, Middx (mimeo).

Churchill, D.N., Morgan, J. and Torrance, G.W. (1984). Cost-effectiveness analysis comparing ambulatory peritoneal dialysis to hospital haemodialysis. *Medical Decision Making*, **4** (4), 489–500.

Craig, T.J., Comstock, G.W. and Geiser, P.B. (1974). The quality of survival in breast cancer: a case control comparison. *Cancer*, **333**, 1451–7.

Drummond, M.F., Stoddart, G.L. and Torrance, G.W. (1987). *Methods for the Economic Evaluation of Health Care Programmes*, Oxford University Press.

Greer, S., Morris, T. and Pettingale, K.W. (1979). Psychological response to breast cancer: effect on outcome. *Lancet*, October 1979, 785–787.

Kind, P., Rosser, R. and Williams, A. (1982). Valuation of quality of life: some psychometric evidence. In Jones-Lee, M.W.(ed.), *The Value of Life and Safety*, Amsterdam: North-Holland, .159–170.

Llewellyn-Thomas, H.A., Sutherland, H.J., Tibshirani, R. *et al.* (1984). Describing health states: methodologic issues in obtaining values for health states. *Medical Care*, **22** (6), 543–52.

Maguire, G.P., Lee, E.G., Bevington, D.J. *et al.* (1978). Psychiatric problems in the first year after mastectomy. *British Medical Journal*, **1**, 963–5.

McNeil, B.J., Weichselbaum, R. and Pauker, S.G. (1981). Trade-offs between quality and quantity of life in laryngeal cancer. *New England Journal of Medicine*, **305** (17), 982–7.

Meyerowitz, B.E., Sparks, F.C. and Spears, I.K. (1983). Adjuvant chemotherapy for breast cancer. *Cancer*, **43**, 1613–8.

Mohide, E.A., Torrance, G.W., Streiner, D.L. *et al.* (1987). *Measuring the Well-being of Family Care Givers Using the Time Trade-off Technique*, Hamilton, Ontario: McMaster University (mimeo).

Morris, T., Greer, H.S. and White, P. *et al.* (1977). Psychological and social adjustment to mastectomy, *Cancer*, **40**, 2381–7.

Neumann, J. von and Morgenstern, O. (1985). *Theory of Games and Economic Behaviour*, 3rd ed, New York: Wiley.

O'Connor, A.M., Boyd, N.F. and Till, J.E. (1985). Influence of elicitation technique, position order and test-retest error on preferences for alternative cancer drug therapy, in *Proceedings of the 10th National Nursing Research Conference*, Toronto: University of Toronto.

Patrick, D.L., Bush, J.W. and Chen, M.M. (1973). Methods for measuring levels of well-being for a health status index, *Health Services Research*, **8** (3), 228–45.

Sackett, D.L. and Torrance, G.W. (1978). The utility of different health states as perceived by the general public, *Journal of Chronic Diseases*, **31** (11), 697–704.

Torrance, G.W. (1976). Social preferences for health states: an empirical evaluation of three measurement techniques, *Socio-Economic Planning Sciences*, **10** (3), 128–36.

Torrance, G.W. (1986). Measurement of health state utilities for economic appraisal: a review, *Journal of Health Economics*, 5, 1–30.

Torrance, G.W. and Mohide, E.A. (1985). *Time Trade-off Instrument: Interview Schedule, Recording Forms and Props*, McMaster University, mimeo, August 1985.

Van Dam, F.S.A., Linssen, A.C.G., Engelsman, E. *et al.* (1980). Life with cytostatic drugs, in *Breast Cancer: Experimental and Clinical Aspects*, Proceedings of the Second EORTC Breast Cancer Working Conference, 229–33.

Winick, L. and Robbins, G.F. (1977). Physical and psychological readjustment after mastectomy, *Cancer*, **39**, 478–86.

Appendix A: Examples of Health State Scenarios Used in the Study

---

Situation L:

Mrs Lewis's Situation

Diagnosed and treated for breast cancer one year ago.

Treated surgically by simple mastectomy—removal of the whole breast followed by plastic surgery to make a new breast.

Occasionally concerned that the cancer will come back.

Feels confident and in control of her life.

Friends and family enjoy visiting and being visited by her.

Interests and hobbies have continued as before diagnosis.

Partner is supportive.

Sexual relations are good.

Situation T:

Mrs Turner's Situation

Diagnosed and treated for breast cancer one year ago.

Treated surgically by simple mastectomy—removal of the whole breast.

Some swelling and stiffness of the arm, requiring looser clothing and restricting movement.

Completely engulfed by fears that the cancer will come back, and of death.

Not able to go out and meet people.

Tearful, does not sleep well.

Very sensitive about her appearance, even when clothed.

Partner is not supportive.

Sexual relations have declined.

Measuring Health: A Practical Approach
Edited by G. Teeling Smith
© 1988 John Wiley & Sons Ltd

6

Assessment of Quality of Life in Parkinson's Disease

Peter Welburn
Janssen Pharmaceutical Ltd., UK

and

Stuart Walker
Centre for Medicines Research, Carshalton, Surrey

Introduction

Parkinson's disease is a crippling, degenerative, neurological condition that affects 60–80,000 people in the UK, the great majority of whom are aged over 60. It presents essentially as a motoric disorder but may lead also to depression and cognitive impairments of varying degrees of seriousness. The disease is mainly a disorder of late life (on average about 65 years), with a sex incidence that is approximately equal.

Symptomatology

Today, Parkinson's disease is recognized as having a classic triad of symptoms; tremor, rigidity and bradykinesia. A rhythmic tremor is perhaps the most recognizable symptom and is said to be the initial symptom in 70 per cent of patients with Parkinson's disease (Hoehn and Yahr, 1967). It is not a continuous tremor, but occurs rather intermittently and is particularly evident when the affected limbs are at rest, or when the patient is concentrating or feeling anxious.

Cogwheel rigidity, the second major symptom, is experienced by patients as muscle stiffness, soreness or cramping. Because the muscles are constantly contracted they may shorten, particularly in the back, drawing the head and neck downward and causing back pain, poor balance, propulsion and falling.

Bradykinesia, the final symptom of the triad, is characterized by a certain slowness of, or even inability to initiate, movement. Fatigue, diminution in automatic movements (e.g., eye blinking and swallowing), a soft monotonous voice, festinating gait, and an immobile 'masked-like' facial expression are examples of bradykinesia. This symptom, like tremor, varies from moment to moment, with the patient still able to perform tasks in a smooth and vigorous manner on some occasions.

A diagnosis of Parkinson's disease is made when there is evidence of all three symptoms, though each component of the triad may vary considerably in its seriousness (Duvoisin, 1984).

Treatment

In his 'Essay on the shaking palsy', James Parkinson (1817) wrote 'until we are better informed, respecting the nature of this disease, the employment of internal medicine is scarcely warranted'. However, over the past 25 years an increased understanding of the disease has resulted and because of this, the control of parkinsonism with modern medicines has progressed rapidly. Today, in the UK, there are five main classes of medicines used to treat Parkinson's disease (Table 1).

Table 1. Drugs currently used in the management of Parkinson's disease

Group	Generic name	Trade name
L-dopa preparations	L-dopa + benserazide	Madopar
	L-dopa + carbidopa	Sinemet
Anticholinergics	Benzhexol	Artane
	Benztropine	Cogentin
	Biperiden	Akineton
	Methixene	Tremonil
	Orphenadrine	Disipal
	Procyclidine	Kemadrin
Others	Amantadine	Symmetrel
	Bromocriptine	Parlodel
	Selegiline	Eldepryl

At all stages of disease severity the treatment has to be related to both the symptoms and the disability (Pearce,1984). It should also be tailored to the patient's need, bearing in mind age, concurrent illness, compliance, the possible coexistence of dementia and the past history of toxicity.

Anticholinergic compounds have been used to treat Parkinson's disease for well over 100 years, and probably act centrally, preventing the action of acetyl choline at receptor sites. They reduce tremor, rigidity and akinesia by about 20 per cent. Side effects (dry mouth, blurred vision and constipation) are particularly common in elderly parkinsonian patients, who are also susceptible to confusional states which may be induced during treatment (Barbeau, 1972).

The antiviral compound, amantidine, is chemically unrelated to other antiparkinsonian compounds. However, its effect in Parkinson's disease is probably related to that of amphetamines, enhancing central dopamine and noradrenaline transmission. It has an additive effect when administered with anticholinergics but its effects tend to be short-lived (Parkes, 1975) and thus it is now seldom used.

Levodopa, coupled with a peripheral dopa-decarboxylase inhibitor (e.g. carbidopa or benserazide) is probably the modern day treatment of choice in Parkinson's disease. These inhibitors prevent the peripheral degradation of levodopa to dopamine thus enabling more of the medicine to enter the brain (Marsden *et al.*, 1973). They reduce rigidity, bradykinesia, freezing and posture, but have a lesser and variable effect on tremor. Improvement is achieved in about 90 per cent of patients who present early and it is claimed that these medicines improve the Quality of Life for most patients, but do not halt disease progression. Concern still exists, however, about their long-term safety and sustained therapy causes a number of disabling and dose-limiting complications. Capricious swings in motor performance, usually due to end-of-dose deterioration, are a disturbing example of levodopa induced effects. On/off fluctuations in response, bearing little relationship to dose or timing of administration, are also common after long-term treatment (Marsden and Parkes, 1976). Induced dyskinesia and dystonia (Shaw *et al.*, 1980; Quinn *et al.*, 1982) and psychiatric symptoms (Marttila and Rinne, 1976; Mayeux *et al.*, 1981) are also important limiting factors in the treatment of Parkinson's disease with levodopa analogues.

Bromocriptine and pergolide are both potent dopamine receptor agonists which have antiparkinsonian action similar to levodopa (Godwin-Austen and Smith, 1977; Lees and Stern, 1981; Lieberman and Goldstein, 1982). Both compounds are most useful in patients with fluctuating on/off responses to levodopa (Hardie *et al.*, 1984). Side-effects are similar to those of levodopa, but psychiatric problems are more severe and may be more protracted. They can occur in younger patients and not necessarily in those with long-standing or severe disability.

Selegiline, a selective type-B monoamine oxidase inhibitor, is probably the most recent approach to the treatment of Parkinson's disease. It potentiates the effects of levodopa and is a useful adjunct in patients exhibiting end-of-dose deterioration, or on/off swings (Stern *et al.*, 1983). Side-effects are not usually a problem, but may include nightmares, postural hypotension, confusion, dizziness and headaches (Brodersen *et al.*, 1985).

Parkinson's Disease and Quality of Life

Parkinson's disease is easily recognized by the onlooker, on account of its basic clinical features, that is, tremor, rigidity, akinesia, postural instability and postural deformity, and as a result, most of the subjective rating scales, and activity of daily living scales developed to assess disease severity, rely heavily on these features.

The first attempt to quantify disease severity was made by Riklan and Diller (1956) who devised a 98-item scale listing various activities of daily living. Unfortunately, this scale proved to be neither reliable nor workable, and is no longer in use. In contrast, the North-Western University Disability Scale (Canter *et al.*, 1961) and the Webster Rating Scale (Webster, 1968) have both been used widely and reliably to assess the signs and symptoms of Parkinsonism. The North-Western University Disability Scale (Appendix 1) consists of a 5- or 10-point rating for walking, dressing, hygiene, feeding and speech, based on clearly defined criteria. In the Webster scale (Appendix 2) bradykinesia of the hands, rigidity, posture, upper extremity swing, gait, tremor, facies, seborrhoea, speech and self-care are all assessed using a 0–3 rating system.

Some investigators have developed combined subjective rating scales with simple objective tests of motor function (Godwin-Austen *et al.*, 1969; Parkes *et al.*, 1970). The most frequently used objective tests involve the use of peg boards, the time taken to put on mittens or socks and the time taken to walk a measured distance. Most of these scales were developed and applied successfully to demonstrate the therapeutic efficacy of levodopa and other antiparkinsonian drugs in the late 1960s and early 1970s.

Perhaps the most popular and simplest method of staging Parkinson's disease was devised by Hoehn and Yahr (1967) (Appendix 3). This scale provides a generally accepted basis for assessing the severity of parkinsonism, and Lieberman *et al.* (1980) have reported a good correlation between the Hoen and Yahr staging and more detailed scoring systems. Unfortunately such staging is relatively insensitive to changes in the patient's clinical state. Hoehn and Yahr also reported a marked discrepancy between the primary signs of Parkinson's disease, such as tremor and rigidity, and the degree of functional incapacity. In fact most patients are less concerned with the severity of rigidity and tremor than they are with the effects of these and other clinical features of the disease, on activities such as walking, dressing and manual dexterity. Also, most patients look upon Parkinson's disease as a progressive and very debilitating illness causing embarrassment, loneliness and depression, with increasing dependence on others, as well as restricting mobility around and outside the home. Hence the psychosocial factors associated with the disease may well be more important in influencing quality of life than are the primary symptoms, and the most recent work on evaluating quality of life in Parkinson's disease has concentrated on these aspects of the disease using patient-rated questionnaires and rating scales.

Bulpitt *et al.* (1985) administered a 61-item questionnaire to a group of patients with Parkinson's disease, and compared their responses with those of a control group, who were randomly selected from a general practice in Harlow near London. Table 2 gives the percentage of the patients and the control subjects complaining of the various symptoms. The symptoms are ordered according to the ratio of patient complaints to control subject complaints. These ratios represent the strength of the association between Parkinson's disease (or its treatment) and the symptoms. The greatest ratios were associated with the complaints of being frozen or rooted to the spot, grimacing, jerking of limbs, and shaking of hands, all classic symptoms of Parkinson's disease.

Table 2. Symptoms with more than a two fold excess in parkinsonian patients compared with controls (from Bulpitt, 1985)

Symptom	Patient group	Control group	Ratio of complaint rates
Frozen or rooted to spot	40.8	1.0	41.0 : 1
Grimacing	39.2	2.0	19.5 : 1
Jerking of arms and legs	46.3	3.0	15.3 : 1
Shaking of hands	61.7	6.0	10.3 : 1
Mouth waters excessively	38.5	4.0	9.8 : 1
Clumsy hands	56.4	6.0	9.3 : 1
Poor concentration	33.1	4.0	8.3 : 1
Severe apprehension	34.5	5.0	7.0 : 1
Hallucinations	17.0	3.0	5.7 : 1
Faintness on standing	54.5	11.8	4.6 : 1

Source: Bulpitt (1985).

Recently, more general quality of life measures, such as the Nottingham Health Profile (NHP) (Hunt and McEwen, 1980) and the Sickness Impact Profile (SIP) (Bergner *et al.*, 1981) have been used to evaluate quality of life in patients with Parkinson's disease.

The NHP is in two parts: Part 1 contains 38 questions describing health problems in six areas; energy, sleep, pain, physical mobility, social isolation and emotions. Part 2 contains 7 statements relating to the effects of health problems on occupation, household management, family life, sex life, social life, holidays and hobbies. The subject responds with 'yes' or 'no' according to whether the statement applies to him/her or not. The statements in Part 1 have been weighted to reflect the fact that the problems vary in severity and each

Peter Welburn and Stuart Walker

of the six sections carries a maximum score of 100. Statements in Part 2 are scored one for a 'yes' response and zero for a 'no' response.

The NHP was chosen initially, as the most suitable of the established quality of life instruments to use in Parkinson's disease for the following reasons:

Previous investigations had demonstrated its sensitivity in a wide range of situations (McEwen, 1983).
Validity and reliability were reported to be high (Backett *et al.*, 1981).
Easy and inexpensive to use and can be self-administered.

The NHP was initially administered to 55 outpatients from the Parkinson's Disease Clinic at King's College Hospital (KCH) in London. Figure 1 illustrates the results obtained from an analysis of the responses to Part 1 of the profile. The patients reported most problems in the areas of energy, physical mobility, emotions and social isolation. Furthermore, when these results are compared with ones obtained from an age-matched group of 'healthy' elderly subjects (randomly selected from a general practice in Twyford) and a group of outpatients with Peripheral Vascular Disease (PVD) it is quite clearly possible to distinguish the three groups on the basis of their response to Part 1 of the NHP.

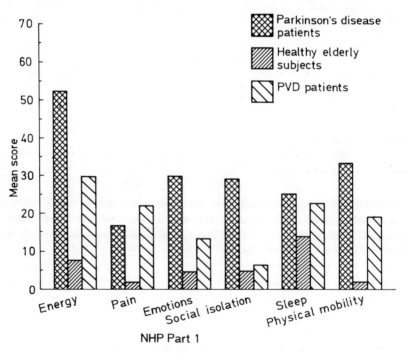

Figure 1. Comparison of the NHP Part 1 scores

In addition to the above areas, communication problems have also been reported by other authors (Oxtoby, 1982; Sutcliffe *et al.*, 1985; Gotham *et al.*, 1986). In these studies patients expressed difficulties in writing a letter and considered that their speech was sometimes unintelligible. In Parkinson's disease, speech is generally lower in volume, higher in pitch, and faster than normal, with a disorder of metred speech rather than errors in articulation (Scott and Caird, 1984). Written communication is also impaired as handwriting becomes difficult, and although many resort to slow writing using a capital script, illegibility is still common. Writing and speech do improve with levodopa (Mawdsley and Gamsu, 1971) but it has been difficult to show whether or not speech therapy is definitely beneficial in the long term. Data which are reported later in the chapter, using the SIP in patients with Parkinson's disease, also highlighted communication as a problem in these patients. Parkinsonian patients also reported problems with walking around indoors without assistance, in the studies conducted by Sutcliffe *et al.* (1985) and Gotham *et al.* (1986).

Other studies have also found a high prevalence of emotional problems, and in particular depression, in patients with Parkinson's disease when compared with other disease states (Mindham, 1970; Robins, 1976; Mayeux *et al.*, 1984). However, attempts to relate the severity of depression to the degree of disability have been unsuccessful, and most studies have shown no significant correlation.

Figure 2 records the results obtained from the responses to Part 2 of the NHP when administered to the KCH Parkinson's disease patients, the 'healthy' elderly subjects and the PVD patients. The parkinsonian patients, in contrast to the other groups, reported most problems with homecare, hobbies, holidays and social life, but all the areas listed in Part 2 were in fact severely affected by the disease. The apparently low response to the 'occupation' statement by the parkinsonian patients is actually a misleading figure as the majority of the patients had already given up work because of the effects of the illness.

Singer (1973) also investigated the effects of parkinsonism on work and income, household management and leisure roles, comparing the results to national norms for an age-matched population. He reported a significant increase in unemployment in the patient group and, in those still working, the number of days lost through illness was much higher than the national average for the same age. Fewer of the patients engaged in housework, while reading and watching television were the most common leisure activities, particularly in the over-65s. A second study, conducted in Glasgow, also assessed the relationship between disease severity, and the curtailment of a patient's hobbies and pastimes (Manson and Caird, 1985). The results indicated that sedentary activities such as reading and watching television were little altered, whereas outdoor activities were markedly affected. Furthermore, few new activities were commenced after the onset of the illness.

In the KCH study, the patients also rated their own health as very good, good, fair, poor or very poor, in addition to completing the NHP (Figure 3).

Peter Welburn and Stuart Walker

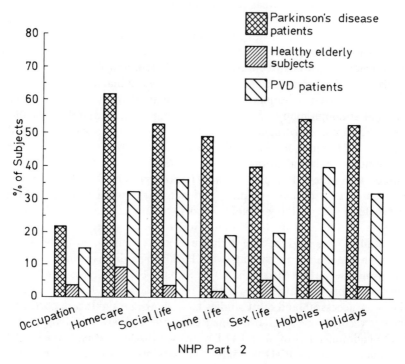

Figure 2. Comparison of the NHP Part 2 scores

Similar responses were also obtained from the 'healthy' elderly subjects and the PVD patients and again the three groups can be clearly distinguished. Table 3 gives the correlations between the NHP Part 1 scores, and the patient-rated health. A strong association can be seen between a number of the sections of Part 1 (physical mobility, emotions and energy) and the patient-rated health. Subset regression analysis of these results revealed that the best subset of NHP Part 1 scores, predictive of the patient-rated health score were: energy, sleep and physical mobility. From these initial results, it was apparent that the NHP could be used to quantify how Parkinson's disease affects a patient's quality of life and thus further studies were warranted. A second study was therefore conducted using a different group of outpatients with Parkinson's disease (Derby Royal Infirmary) to compare the NHP with the Sickness Impact Profile (SIP) (Bergner *et al.*, 1981).

The SIP is a self-administered measure of sickness-related dysfunction, which consists of 12 categories of activity: Ambulation (A), Mobility (M), Body Control and Movement (BCM), Social Interaction (SI), Communication (C), Alertness Behaviour (AB), Emotional Behaviour (EB), Sleep and Rest (SR), Eating (E), Home Management (HM), Recreation and Pastimes (RP) and Work (W).

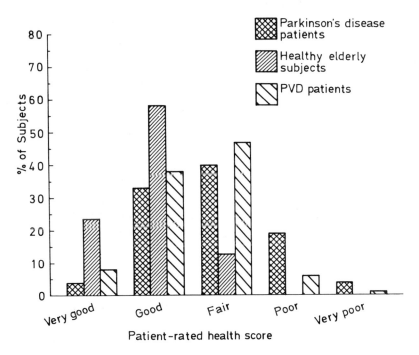

Figure 3. Comparison of the patient-rated health scores

Table 3. Correlations between NHP Part 1 scores and patient-rated health

	Patient-rated health	Energy	Pain	Emotions	Sleep	Social isolation	Physical mobility
Patient-rated health	1.00						
Energy	0.43	1.00					
Pain	0.23	0.47	1.00				
Emotions	0.46	0.67	0.55	1.00			
Sleep	0.10	0.49	0.43	0.62	1.00		
Social isolation	0.30	0.39	0.27	0.67	0.64	1.00	
Physical mobility	0.57	0.51	0.60	0.67	0.38	0.44	1.00

All items for each subscale are assigned a weighted value, summed, and then divided by the total possible subscale score. This ratio is then multiplied by 100 to give a percentage dysfunction score for each of the twelve categories.

In addition to the separate subscale scores, summary scores are also provided for physical dysfunction (derived from Ambulation, Mobility and Body Control and Movement subscales) and psychosocial dysfunction (derived from Social Interaction, Communication, Alertness Behaviour and Emotional Behaviour subscales). An overall score can also be derived from all 12 subscales yielding an index for quality of life.

Forty-five parkinsonian patients in total completed both the NHP and the SIP, by mail, in randomized fashion, two months apart. Preliminary results from this second study, illustrated in Figures 4 and 5, quite clearly demonstrate the similarity of the category scores from the NHP, for different populations of the same disease group. It also confirms the flexibility in the method of administration of the profile. Furthermore, patient-rated health was also very similar for both groups of patients with Parkinson's disease (Figure 6).

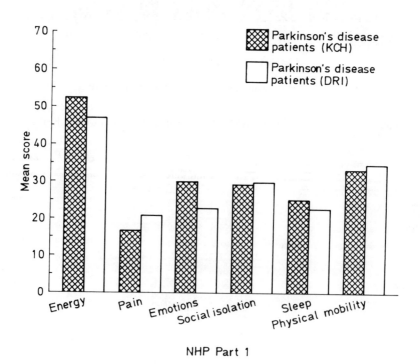

Figure 4. Comparison of the NHP Part 1 scores

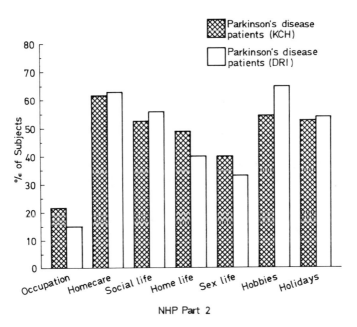

Figure 5. Comparison of the NHP Part 2 scores

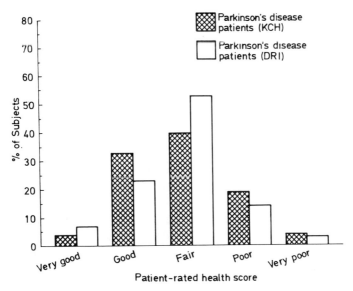

Figure 6. Comparison of the patient-rated health scores

Analysis of the SIP data from this study is illustrated in Figure 7. As was seen with the NHP, patients reported most problems (highest per cent Dysfunction Scores) in the areas of Home Management, Communication, Alertness Behaviour, Ambulation and Recreation and Pastimes, with Eating and Work being the areas least affected. The results on Eating were unexpected; the majority of patients with long-standing Parkinson's disease have great difficulty in handling eating utensils and hence it would have been expected that this would reflect adversely on eating. This apparent anomaly is currently being investigated further. Figure 7 also compares the SIP data from the parkinsonian patients with data published by Klonoff *et al.* (1986) for patients two to four years after Closed Head Injury (CHI). As was seen with the NHP and the PVD patients, the parkinsonian patients scored much higher than the CHI patients and the SIP was capable of distinguishing between the two groups.

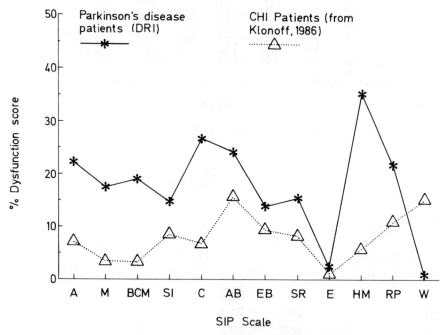

Figure 7. Comparison of the SIP % Dysfunction Scores

Table 4 lists the Physical Dysfunction summary score, the Psychosocial Dysfunction summary score and the overall SIP score for the parkinsonian patients, the CHI patients and a group of disabled patients reported by Charlton *et al.*, (1983). Again the results demonstrate that the SIP is capable of quantifying the devastating effect Parkinson's disease has on a patient's quality of life, as measured by these three summary scores.

Table 4. Physical Dysfunction summary scores, Psychosocial Dysfunction summary scores, and the Overall SIP scores

Patient group	Physical dysfunction score	Psychosocial dysfunction score	Overall SIP score
Parkinson's disease patients	19.42	18.92	18.04
CHI patients (Klonoff, 1986)	3.92	11.09	9.59
Disabled patients (Charlton, 1983)	13.06	15.65	11.84

Conclusions

From the results of these initial studies it has been demonstrated that Parkinson's disease does severely affect certain aspects of a patient's life, and that these effects can be quantified by using either the NHP or the SIP. Further studies are now needed to explore the correlation between patient-rated disease severity as measured by either the NHP or the SIP, and disease severity as measured by one of the physician-rated disability scales. Longitudinal studies are also required to demonstrate the reproducibility of these instruments over time, and before and during treatment. The NHP and SIP could also be usefully employed in the future evaluation of new therapies for the treatment of Parkinson's disease, and perhaps one day play a role in helping decide the most appropriate treatment to prescribe, for a particular patient.

References

Backett, E.M. *et al*. (1981). Health and Quality of Life—end of grant report No. HR 6157/1. London: Social Science Research Council.

Barbeau, A. (1972). *Neurology*, **22**, 22.

Bergner, M. *et al*. (1981). The Sickness Impact Profile: Development and final revision of a Health Status Measure. *Medical Care*, **29**, 787–805.

Brodersen, P. *et al*. (1985). The effect of L-deprenyl on the on/off phenomena in Parkinson's disease. *Acta Neurol. Scand*., **71**, 494.

Bulpitt, C.J. *et al*. (1985). The symptoms of patients treated for Parkinson's disease. *Clin. Neuropharmacol*., **8**, 175–83.

Canter, C.J. *et al*. (1961). A method of evaluating disability in patients with Parkinson's disease. *J. nerve. mental. Dis*., **133**, 143–7.

Duvoisin, R.C. (1984). Parkinson's Disease: A guide for patient and family (2nd edn.), New York: Raven Press.

Godwin-Austen, R.B. *et al*. (1969). Effects of L-dopa in Parkinson's disease. *Lancet*, **2**, 165.

Godwin-Austen, R.B. and Smith, N.J. (1977). Comparison of the effects of bromocriptine and levodopa in Parkinson's disease. *J. Neurol. Neurosurg. Psychiat*., **40**, 479.

Gotham, A.M. *et al*. (1986). Depression in Parkinson's disease: a quantitative and qualitative analysis. *J. Neurol. Neurosurg. Psychiat*., **49**, 38–9.

Hardie, R.J. *et al.*, (1984). On–off fluctuations in Parkinson's disease. A clinical and neuropharmacological study. *Brain*, **107**, 487.

Hoehn, M.M. and Yahr, M.D. (1967). Parkinsonism: onset, progression and mortality. *Neurology*, **17**, 427.

Hunt, S.M. and McEwen, J. (1980). The development of a Subjective Health Indicator. *Sociology of Health and Illness*, **2**(3), 231.

Klonoff, P.S. *et al.* (1986). Quality of Life in Patients 2 to 4 Years after Closed Head Injury. *Neurosurgery*, **19**, 735.

Lees, A.J. and Stern, G.M. (1981). Pergolide and lisuride for levodopa induced oscillations. *Lancet*, **II**, 577.

Lieberman, A. *et al.* (1980). Evaluation of Parkinson's disease. In *Ergot Compounds and Brain Function: neuroendocrine and neuropsychiatric aspects*, ed. Goldstein, M. New York: Raven Press, p. 277.

Lieberman, A. and Goldstein, M. (1982). Treatment of advanced Parkinson's disease with dopamine agonists. In *Movement Disorders*, ed. Marsden, C.D. and Fahn, S. London: Butterworths, p. 146.

Manson, L. and Caird, F.I. (1985). Survey of the hobbies and transport of patients with Parkinson's disease. *Occ. Ther.*, **199**.

Marsden, C.D. *et al.* (1973). A year's comparison of treatment of patients with Parkinson's disease with levodopa versus treatment with levodopa alone. *Lancet*, **II**, 1459.

Marsden, C.D. and Parkes, J.D. (1976). On-off effects in patients with Parkinson's disease on chronic levodopa. *Lancet*, **I**, 292.

Marttila, R.J. and Rinne, U.K. (1976). Dementia in Parkinson's Disease. *Acta Neurol. Scand.*, **54**, 431.

Mawdsley, C. and Gamsu, C.V. (1971). Periodicity of speech in Parkinson's disease. *Nature*, **231**, 315.

Mayeux, R. *et al.* (1981). Depression, intellectual impairment and Parkinson's disease. *Neurology*, **31**, 645.

Mayeux, R. *et al.* (1984). Altered serotonin metabolism in depressed patients with Parkinson's disease. *Neurology*, **34**, 642.

McEwen, J. (1983). The Nottingham health profile. In *Measuring the Social Benefits of Medicines*, ed. Teeling-Smith, G. London: OHE, p. 75.

Mindham, R.H.S. (1970). Psychiatric symptoms in parkinsonism. *J. Neurol. Neurosurg. Psychiat.*, **33**, 188.

Oxtoby, M. (1982). Parkinson's disease patients and their social needs. Parkinson's Disease Society publication.

Parkes, J.D. *et al.* (1970). Amantadine dosage in the treatment of Parkinson's disease. *Lancet*, **I**, 1130.

Parkes, J.D. (1975). *Advances in Drug Research*, **8**, 11.

Parkinson, J. (1817). *An Essay on the Shaking Palsy*. London: Sherwood, Neely and Jones.

Pearce, J.M.S. (1984). Drug treatment of Parkinson's disease. *Brit. Med. J.*, **288**, 1777.

Quinn, N. *et al.* (1982). Complicated response fluctuations in Parkinson's disease: response to intravenous infusion of levodopa. *Lancet*, **II**, 412.

Riklan, M. and Diller, L. (1956). Certain psychomotor aspects of subtemporal pallidectomy for Parkinson's disease. *J. Am. Geriat. Soc.*, **4**, 1258.

Robins, A.H. (1976). Depression in patients with parkinsonism. *Brit. J. Psychiat.*, **128**, 141.

Scott, S. and Caird, F.I. (1984). The response of the apparent receptive speech disorder of Parkinson's disease to speech therapy. *J. Neurol. Neurosurg. Psychiat.*, **47**, 302.

Shaw, K.M. *et al*. (1980). The impact of treatment with levodopa on Parkinson's disease. *Quart. J. Med.*, **49**, 283.

Stern, G.M. *et al*. (1983). *Acta. Neurol. Scand.*, **95**(suppl), 113.

Sutcliffe, R.L. *et al*. (1985) Parkinson's disease in the district of the Northampton Health Authority (UK): a study of prevalence and disability. *Acta. Neurol. Scand.*, **72**, 363.

Webster, D.D. (1968). Clinical analysis of the disability in Parkinson's disease. *Mod. Treat.*, **5**, 257.

Appendix 1: North-Western University Disability Scale

Scale A: Walking

Never walks alone.

0. Cannot walk at all, even with maximum assistance
1. Needs considerable help, even for short distances, cannot walk outdoors without help
2. Requires moderate help indoors; walks outdoors with considerable help
3. Requires potential help indoors and active help outdoors
4. Walks from room to room without assistance, but moves slowly and uses external support; never walks alone outdoors
5. Walks from room to room with only moderate difficulty; may occasionally walk outdoors without assistance
6. Walks short distances with ease; walking outdoors is difficult but often accomplished without help
7. Gait is extremely abnormal; very slow and shuffling; posture grossly affected; there may be propulsion
8. Quality of gait is poor and rate is slow; posture moderately affected; there may be a tendency towards mild propulsion; turning is difficult
9. Gait only slightly deviant from normal in quality and speed; turning is the most difficult task; posture essentially normal
10. Normal

Scale B: Dressing

Requires complete assistance

0. Patient is a hindrance rather than a help to assistant
1. Movements of patient neither help nor hinder assistant
2. Can give some help through bodily movements
3. Gives considerable help through bodily movements
4. Performs only gross dressing activities alone (hat, coat)
5. Performs about half of dressing activities independently
6. Performs more than half of dressing activities alone, with considerable effort and slowness

7. Handles all dressing alone with the exception of fine activities (tie, buttons)
8. Dresses self completely with slowness and great effort
9. Dresses self completely with only slightly more time and effort than normal
10. Normal

Scale C: Hygiene

Requires complete assistance

0. Unable to maintain proper hygiene even with maximum help
1. Reasonably good hygiene with assistance, but does not provide assistant with significant help
2. Hygiene maintained well; gives aid to assistant, requires partial assistance
3. Performs a few tasks alone with assistant nearby
4. Requires assistance for half of toilet needs
5. Requires assistance for some tasks not difficult in terms of co-ordination
6. Manages most of personal needs alone; has substituted methods for accomplishing difficult tasks. Complete self-help
7. Hygiene maintained independently, but with effort and slowness; accidents are not infrequent; may employ substitute methods
8. Hygiene activities are moderately time-consuming; no substitute methods; few accidents
9. Hygiene maintained normally; with exception of slight slowness
10. Normal

Scale D: Eating and Feeding (scored separately)

Eating

0. Eating is so impaired that a hospital setting is required to get adequate nutrition
1. Eats only soft foods and liquids; these are consumed very slowly
2. Liquids and soft foods handled with ease; hard foods occasionally eaten, but require great effort and much time
3. Eats some hard foods routinely, but these require time and effort
4. Follows a normal diet, but chewing and swallowing are laboured
5. Normal

Feeding

0. Requires complete assistance
1. Performs only few feeding tasks independently
2. Performs most feeding tasks alone, slowly and with effort, requires help with feeding

3. Handles all feeding alone with moderate slowness, still may get assistance in specific situation (e.g. cutting meat in restaurant); accidents are not infrequent
4. Fully feeds self with rare accidents; slower than normal
5. Normal

Scale E: Speech

0. Does not vocalize at all
1. Vocalizes, but rarely for communicative purposes
2. Vocalizes to call attention to self
3. Attempts to use speech for communication, but has difficulty in initiating vocalism; may stop speaking in middle of phrase and be unable to continue
4. Uses speech in most communication, but articulation is highly unintelligible; may have occasional difficulty in initiating speech; usually speaks in single words or short phrases
5. Speech always employed for communication, but articulation is still very poor, usually uses complete sentences
6. Speech can always be understood if listener pays close attention; both articulation and voice may be defective
7. Communication accomplished with ease, although speech impairments detract from content
8. Speech easily understood, but voice or speech rhythm may be disturbed
9. Speech entirely adequate; minor voice disturbances present
10. Normal

Appendix 2: Webster's Parkinson's disease rating scale

Directions

Apply a gross clinical rating to each of the 10 listed items, assigning value ratings of 0–3 for each item, where (0) = no involvement and (1), (2) and (3) are equated to early, moderate and severe disease respectively

Bradykinesia of hands (including handwriting)

(0) No involvement
(1) Detectable lowering of the pronation-supination rate, evidenced by beginning of difficulty in handling tools, buttoning clothes and with handwriting
(2) Moderate slowing of supination-pronation rate, one or both sides, evidenced by moderate impairment of hand function. Handwriting is greatly impaired, micrographia is present
(3) Severe slowing of supination-pronation rate. Unable to write or button clothes. Marked difficulty in handling utensils

Rigidity

(0) None detectable
(1) Detectable rigidity in neck and shoulders. Activation[1] phenomenon is present. One or both arms show mild, negative[2] resting rigidity
(2) Moderate rigidity in neck and shoulders. Resting rigidity is positive[2] when patient not on medication
(3) Severe rigidity in neck and shoulders. Resting rigidity cannot be reversed by medication

Posture

(0) Normal Posture. Head flexed forward less than 4 inches
(1) Beginning 'poker' spine. Head flexed forward up to 5 inches
(2) Beginning arm flexion. Head flexed forward up to 6 inches. One or both arms raised but still below the waist
(3) Onset of simian posture. Head flexed forward more than 6 inches. One or both hands elevated above the waist. Sharp flexion of hand, beginning interphalangeal extension. Beginning flexion of knees

Upper extremity swing

(0) Swings both arms well
(1) Gait shortened to 12–18 inch stride. Beginning to strike one heel. Turn around time slowing. Requires several steps
(2) Stride moderately shortened, now 6–12 inches. Both heels beginning to strike floor forcefully
(3) Onset of shuffling gait, steps less than 3 inches. Occasional stuttering type of blocking gait. Walks on toes—turns around very slowly

Tremor

(0) None detectable
(1) Less than 1 inch of peak-to-peak tremor movement observed in limbs or head at rest or in either hand while walking or during finger to nose testing
(2) Maximum tremor envelope fails to exceed 4 inches. Tremor is severe but not constant and patient retains some control of hands
(3) Tremor envelope exceeds 4 inches. Tremor is constant and severe. Patient cannot get free of tremor while awake. Writing and feeding are impossible

---

[1] Activation phenomenon is an increase in rigidity in involved limb evoked by voluntary movement of contralateral limb.
[2] Negative rigidity indicates that the patient aids passive movements performed by the observer, to a greater or lesser extent. Positive rigidity implies involuntary resistance associated with increased tone.

Facies

(0) Normal. Full animation. No stare
(1) Detectable immobility. Mouth remains closed. Beginning features of anxiety and depression
(2) Moderate immobility. Emotion breaks through at markedly increased threshold. Lips parted some of the time. Moderate appearance of anxiety or depression. drooling may be present
(3) Frozen facies. Mouth open 1/4 inch or more. Drooling may be severe

Seborrhoea

(0) None
(1) Increased perspiration. Secretion remaining thin
(2) Obvious oiliness present. Secretion much thicker
(3) Marked seborrhoea, entire face and head covered by thick secretion

Speech

(0) Loud, clear, resonant, easily understood
(1) Beginning of hoarseness with loss of inflection and resonance. Good volume and still easily understood
(2) Moderate hoarseness and weakness. Constant monotone, unvaried pitch. Beginning of dysarthria, hesitancy, stuttering, difficult to understand
(3) Marked hoarseness and weakness. Very difficult to hear and understand

Self-care

(0) No impairment
(1) Still provides full self-care but rate of dressing definitely impaired
(2) Requires help in certain critical areas, such as turning in bed, rising from chairs etc. Very slow in performing most activities, but manages by taking more time
(3) Continuously disabled. Unable to dress, feed or walk alone

Appendix 3: Hoehn and Yahr's (1967) Staging for Parkinson's Disease

Stage I

Unilateral involvement, usually minimal or no functional impairment

Stage II

Bilateral or mid-line involvement, without impairment of balance

Stage III

First signs of impaired righting reflexes; evident in unsteadiness as the patient turns or demonstrated when he is pushed from standing equilibrium with feet together and eyes closed. Functionally somewhat restricted, but may be able to work, depending on nature of employment. Capable of independent living, with mild to moderate overall disability

Stage IV

Fully developed, severely disabling disease. Can stand and walk unaided, but is markedly incapacitated

Stage V

Confined to wheelchair or bed without assistance

Measuring Health: A Practical Approach
Edited by G. Teeling Smith
© 1988 John Wiley & Sons Ltd

7

Assessment of Treatment in Cancer

H. Schipper
*Manitoba Cancer Treatment & Research Foundation,
Winnipeg, Canada*

and

J. Clinch
*Research and Planning Directorate, Manitoba Health,
Winnipeg, Canada*

The purpose of this chapter is to overview, in an evolutionary context, approaches to outcome analysis in clinical cancer. A 'snapshot' overview of cancer outcome analysis techniques fails to take into account the enormous evolution both in the treatment of the medical aspects of malignant disease, and in the social, economic and ethical growth of the communities in which these advances are taking place. There has been an explosion in cancer therapy over the past half-century, based on substantial amounts of progress and promise. Our initial attempts to attack the disease were rewarded by evidence that we could change tumours. We could make them shrink. We could change their growth rates. Occasionally we were able to make them go away. More recently the challenge has been to convert these observations representing a change in the natural history of a tumour into evidence of either remission or cure. Had the goal of cure not been so difficult to achieve, the current evolution to a focus increasingly on quality of outcome would be less intense. Thus, if at the end of this discourse the reader has some sense not only of technique but of direction, the authors' goal will have been achieved.

A Point of Departure

This overview of outcomes and analysis in cancer will focus on the clinical trial. We do so because therapies are generally extrapolated into the community from clinical trials conducted either in a single centre or by multi-institutional groups. It is of course essential in making this therapeutic extrapolation to keep in mind that patients seen in the community may be socially and biologically different from those having the same 'disease' treated in the trial (Hunter *et al.*, 1987). Treatments moved into the community from experimental settings are frequently modified in drug dosage, toxicity attenuation and in characteristics of follow-up, all of which may alter the expected therapeutic outcome. There are few systematic studies of this technology transfer, but such that are available suggest that differences are considerably greater than initially anticipated.

While treatment studies for cancer can be traced back to the ancient Egyptians, the modern clinical trials approach began in the late 1940s and early 1950s with the work of Farber *et al.* (1948) in the treatment of acute lymphoblastic leukaemia of childhood. From the initial observation that folate was an essential co-factor in the metabolism of leukaemia cells came the first clinical trials of a folate antagonist. Partial remissions were readily obtained, very occasionally lasting several months. There followed a series of clinical trials, over two decades, each building on the success of the antecedent trial by asking an additional biological question based on prior observation. Thus when a number of medicines in addition to the antifoles were found to be able to induce transient remission, trials investigating the role of combination therapy were initiated (Henderson, 1967). In so doing occasional transient remissions, followed by marrow and peripheral blood relapse, were converted into longer term remissions where principal sites of failure began to include sequestered sites within the central nervous system (Evans *et al.*, 1970). The next clinical trials addressed this problem with varying combinations of higher dose chemotherapy, intrathecal administration and radiotherapy (Medical Research Council, 1973). The results of these studies were that the CNS relapse rate fell from 30–40 per cent to 5–10 per cent, with a pattern of recurrence shifting again, this time to delayed marrow relapse, other sequestered sites such as the testes, and the development of secondary neoplasia. To address these biological issues further trials asked questions about duration of therapy, the role of marrow transplantation and even more radical radiotherapeutic approaches. Meanwhile two-year survivals had gone from 10 per cent in 1956 to more than 80 per cent in 1976.

As a means of evaluating this data the randomized clinical trials process evolved over twenty years in an attempt to ensure comparability of patients, consistency of patient evaluation and reliability and validity of the mathematical analysis of the data. In overviewing these trials and similar studies leading to the evolution of curative therapies for Hodgkin's Disease (Canellos, 1973; Slayton, 1984), choriocarcinoma and testicular tumours (Garnick, 1985), it is essential to be aware that their success owes to the fortuitous concurrence of a number of biological and statistical conditions:

1. Each new therapy applied had an independent and substantive antitumour effect.
2. The time to the observation of the treatment effect and treatment failure was short.
3. Treatment failure led to death in a short time.
4. Each step in the evolution of therapy led to significant new biological observations about the natural history of the disease, which were directly amenable to a new therapeutic approach.
5. The overall treatment course was short, making it acceptable to use an acute disease model for treatment planning.
6. At most steps along the route, survival differences were considerable, and where they were not, the change in the natural history of disease made clear therapeutic trials possible.

In cancer therapy our dramatic successes are few. For the most part we are faced with common diseases, individual therapies of marginal effectiveness and expected improvements from new therapies which are so small that we are forced to use larger clinical trial designs in order to have the power to detect with confidence such small improvements as may be present. It is in this setting that a refocusing of our endpoints becomes critical. Further, our biological understanding of the disease has to shift from that of an acute illness model, to a more appropriate chronic formulation of the disease.

Intrinsic to the acute leukaemia paradigm is the observation that the natural history of this disease is short. Like a myocardial infarction, the clinical outcome of the disease and its treatment is either survival or death. The outcome is determined in hours, days or short weeks. In such a setting it is appropriate to set aside broader human issues such as economics, social interaction, the family and psychological state. However, for the most part cancer is a chronic disease in which there are remissions and exacerbations, to a greater or lesser extent amenable to therapy. The natural history of the chronic cancers ranges from six months for aggressive small cell carcinomas of the lung to ten to twenty years for some breast cancers and indolent lymphomas. In this setting the fundamental assumptions of the acute care model, namely that the medical aspects of the disease are paramount for short-term therapy, are no longer tenable. Whereas in an acute disease setting patient and physician goals of therapy are likely to be the same, when the disease is both chronic and possibly incurable, therapeutic indicators of success for the physician and the patient may differ. The physician is interested in objective measures of tumour response, as predictors of long-term survival. The patient is concerned with a Gestalt representing quality of life in the context of limited survival. The current interest in 'quality of life' as an outcome measure in cancer trials seeks to bridge the gap between the physician-scientist with his more objective view of outcomes, and the patient with his 'unscientific' personal point of view (Schipper, 1983). The interest is also stimulated by economic concerns relating to the immense cost of current cancer therapies; ethical concerns about limiting therapy in the face of a large array of minimally effective treatments; and social and legal concerns about the changing relationship between patient and physician in the health care scheme (Brown, 1987; Pearlman and Jonsen, 1985; Arora *et al.*, 1986; Thomasma, 1986; Edlund and Tancredi, 1985). Thus what follows is an overview of current standard outcome measures and a more critical review of the emerging quality of life methodologies in order that the reader may find some assistance in designing and carrying out cancer clinical trials, interpreting other clinical trials, and extrapolating from these trials to patient care in the community.

Contemporary Outcome Measures: Phase I, Phase II and Phase III Trials

The assessment of patient outcome in cancer treatment has focused on tumour response, disease-free interval, patient survival and toxicity. Each of these measures has been investigated using one or more of the following different types of studies.

Phase I studies determine the relationship between acute toxic effects and intensity of treatment. New medicines are developed in the laboratory based on biochemical principles and are tested on animals to determine their antitumour effectiveness and toxicity. A usual starting dose for human studies is based on one-tenth of the LD_{10} (the dose which kills 10 per cent of animals treated) in the mouse (Homan, 1972). Patients used in these studies have usually been extensively pre-treated, which may prejudice assessment of tumour response, hence the purpose of these studies is not to determine antitumour effectiveness but to determine only the toxicity of the treatment. Doses are escalated in consecutive sets of patients, often using a modified Fibonacci series (Carter *et al.*, 1977), until a maximally tolerated treatment intensity is determined. Since toxicity is the issue in Phase I trials, the body systems which are anticipated to be the target of the toxic effects should be competent in all patients entered into the trial.

Phase II studies attempt to identify the tumour types which respond to a specific treatment. The outcome measure in this case is the extent of tumour shrinkage observed. Since any change in tumour size is dependent on the measurement technique and its associated human error, criteria for tumour response need to be rigidly defined. Further information on toxicity may be obtained in Phase II trials and related to tumour response.

Often patients entered into Phase II trials have been pre-treated because of the ethical problem of withholding the best existing treatment. For certain types of advanced disease there is no known treatment which prolongs survival and in these cases patients who have received no previous therapy may be used. Pre-treatment builds resistance and therefore such trials will be biased against finding new treatments to be effective (Carter and Selaway, 1977). Consequently these trials must look for a small percentage of responders and have sufficient numbers for power adequate to detect such small response rates.

A two-stage method of determining response rate was suggested by Gehan (1961) based on the binomial distribution. An anticipated response rate is selected and the number of patients that should produce one response with no less than 95 per cent probability is determined. For example, if the true response rate is 10 per cent, then 29 patients should produce at least one responder on no less than 95 per cent of occasions. If the first 29 patients do not show a response the trial is abandoned. If a response is obtained by the time 29 patients have been treated, then additional patients must be treated to obtain a precise estimate of the actual response rate.

New therapies are not likely to be equally effective in the treatment of different histological tumour types and therefore each type should be assessed separately for its response to a new therapy. As both pre-treatment and tumour type will influence response rate, patients should be stratified by both variables when assessing response to the new drug.

Phase III studies are usually comparative in that they determine the effectiveness of a specific treatment in relation to either the natural history of the disease or standard therapy. The usual outcome measures are disease-free interval and survival, but toxicity and tumour response may be reassessed (Figure 1).

Three different types of control group can be used in a Phase III trial, but not all are equally useful. The duration of a trial may be greatly reduced by using historical controls, that is, patients having the same disease who were treated prior to the development of the therapy to be tested. Unfortunately such a design is open to biases no matter how careful one is to avoid them. Patients in the control group were not treated at the same time as patients in the new treatment group, and aspects of their therapy other than the one of interest may have been different. Even though the same selection criteria may have been applied there may be subtle differences in patient selection which go unrecognized. Different physicians entering patients into the trial may well have interpreted and applied the selection criteria in a different manner. The only way to be sure that patients in the treatment and control groups are equivalent is to assign them randomly to their group after selection. Random assignment does not assure that the groups are exactly equal in all other respects except

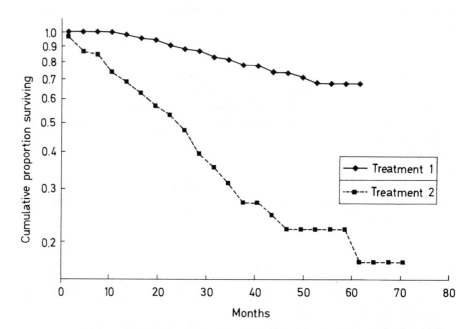

Figure 1.   A typical Phase III clinical trial result. By convention the presentation is a proportion of patients surviving (or disease-free), plotted logarithmically against time. A straight line implies constant risk of recurrence. Note that the curves are monotonically decreasing

the treatment difference of interest, but does allow the specification of an exact probability of them showing outcome differences by chance alone.

Usually the control group in a randomized study receives the previous most effective treatment but occasionally a case can be made for a 'no treatment' arm. If a disease is uniformly and rapidly fatal regardless of any known treatment then it is obviously ethical to use a 'no treatment' arm in the trial. However, there is a natural reluctance to do nothing, even when treatment is toxic, which means that very few randomized studies have 'no treatment' arms.

Phase I and II studies answer narrowly focused questions dealing with separate aspects of patients' response to therapy, whereas Phase III studies answer questions related to their overall response. Thus it is in the context of Phase III trials that quality of life assessment is most relevant. Such assessments have the potential to determine the utility of the trade-offs between the relatively long-term toxic effects of treatment and the duration of survival, that is, between quality and quantity of survival.

There are several important considerations in the organization of a typical Phase III clinical trial:

1. *Patient Selection.* The type of patient eligible for a particular trial must be clearly defined in as much detail as possible. If there are known prognostic factors which influence the course of the disease and its treatment then these must be assessed in each patient selected.
2. *Treatment Protocol.* An exact prescription for the course of treatment in all of the arms of the trial must be defined and all differences except the salient one should be eliminated. Procedures to be adopted in the case of toxic episodes must be outlined and care taken to apply them equally in all treatment groups.
3. *Randomization.* This is the preferred method of treatment assignment because it is the only method of allowing for the presence of unknown factors which influence the progress and outcome of a disease. If a number of prognostic factors are known already, then a stratified randomization should be performed to ensure their equal distribution over the treatment groups.
4. *Sample Size.* This should be calculated to provide sufficient power to detect a specified difference between treatment groups on the chosen outcome variable(s). The smaller the predicted treatment differences, the larger the within-group variability, and the larger the desired power, the larger will be the required sample size. Tables are available for the determination of sample size (Cohen, 1977) for a specified power provided the investigator can determine the effect size of interest. Effect size is the difference in means of the outcome variable between two treatment groups divided by its population standard deviation. When the latter quantity is not known it is possible to use average effect sizes for a particular type of variable which were found from reviews of standard journal articles.

These clinical trial formats focus on outcome measures or endpoints which are considered objective in so far as they are based on external observation of the patient. However, there are a number of factors which may introduce considerable inaccuracy in outcome measures. Warr (1984) has shown, not unexpectedly, that physicians show greater error in determining tumour size the smaller the size of the tumour. Also the estimation of tumour size from X-ray films depends upon the setting of the X-ray machine when the films were taken. Both these types of error can lead to incorrect conclusions that a tumour is shrinking, has disappeared, remained the same size or become larger when in fact one of the other possibilities is correct.

Disease-free interval is also subject to error depending on how often patients are checked for recurrence and upon how closely and exhaustively they are investigated. Even survival time is subject to error. Decisions must be made regarding the starting point for measuring; whether the patient who is now dead was deceased at the time the study follow-up ended; whether a patient's data should be included if death resulted from causes other than the disease or its treatment; what to do with those patients who were lost to follow-up; and the effect of life-support measures on the duration of survival.

In the end, the carefully designed, well-conducted randomized trial may provide statistical evidence of an outcome difference. However, the evidence is mathematical. It remains the obligation of the researcher to assure that the 'significance' has biological and human importance.

An Introduction to the Quality of Life Concept

Quality of life is a rubric which until recently lacked definition. It is a patient-centred concern which has led to a new generation of more subjective measures focusing on patient functional outcome. To date there is no firm consensus about the about the meaning of the term (De Haes and Van Knippenberg, 1985; Calman, 1984; Cribb, 1985; Landesman, 1986; Edlund and Tancredi, 1985; Warr, 1984). Further, the theoretical construct which is usually necessary to the development of a useful test of any form is for the most part lacking, both for test instruments and for the clinical trials in which these measures are employed.

The long argued debate; medicine as art vs medicine as science is rephrased in the conceptual evolution of quality of life. If one views medicine as applied biology, quality of life is a patient-centred final outcome measure, representing one extreme of the applicability of the Scientific Method. At the laboratory level, the physical chemist conducts experiments in a setting that is controllable and repeatable. The tenets of the Scientific Method can be achieved with relatively straightforward identification of significant variables, firm control of dependent and independent variables and considerable precision in measurement. The scientist can be the dispassionate observer. As one moves through single cell systems to organ systems and animal studies it is more difficult to identify and control variables. The multifactorial nature of the biological process makes cause and effect harder to relate, and this difficulty is reflected in broadened criteria for statistical inference, and less certainty in the attribution of cause. Contemporary clinical trials strain the Scientific Method to its limits because of the constraints which derive from applying treatments to a heterogeneous group of people who in the free living state are not biologically controllable. The accuracy of our measurements is constrained by the limits of invasive procedures. In addition, the Heisenberg Uncertainty Principle of physics, that the measurement process itself influences what is being measured, applies in clinical medicine. A diagnostic intervention may itself alter the conditions of the experiment. The best we have been able to do to satisfy strict scientific criteria is to seek objective measures such as survival, disease-free survival and tumour response as endpoints on which to base our experimental conclusions.

In moving to a quality of life measure potentially one gains a major strength; this measure represents the final common pathway of all interventions impinging upon the patient who has cancer. However, to a considerable extent it is subjective. The observer, namely the patient, is not a dispassionate third party. As a final common pathway measure of outcome it can be profoundly influenced by a range of factors not to date considered in trial entry and stratification. For example patient quality of life may be severely impaired by lack of social support (Wortman and Dunkel-Scheiter, 1979). If at the same time as major anticancer therapy is initiated, significant social assistance is provided, a patient's quality of life may improve. To attribute this improvement to the cancer therapy may be misleading.

While a uniformly accepted definition of quality of life has thus far proved elusive, certain important factors which influence the definition have become clear:

1. Who defines quality of life? Physician-scientists are more comfortable when measurements of patient outcome are made by dispassionate third parties. Thus, from this perspective, quality of life represents some aggregation of externally observable parameters such as the ability to return to work, income, or physiological measurements such as PO_2 or haemoglobin. The social scientist is more interested in issues such as social interaction and psychological state. Patients' definitions of quality of life tend to be daily-function orientated, and where elucidated reflect differences between expectation and achievement, satisfaction, hope, etc. (Presant, 1984).
2. The motivation of the observer profoundly affects the definition as well. An economist looking at quality of life focuses on issues of dollar cost for quantum of benefit. Williams' Quality Of Life Equivalent Year (QALY) represents such an econometric model.
3. For issues of life and death, particularly for the unborn or the economically and mentally disadvantaged, quality of life is often blurred with another concept, namely sanctity of life. This leads to the argument that unless a true intellectual discussion of alternatives can be provided, one must assume that the maximum quality of life is synonymous with maximum preservation of life (Edlund and Tancredi, 1985).
4. Unless very great care is taken, the ambient cultural setting will be a major determinant of quality of life. If quality of life is defined against some absolute external standard such as number of hours worked, amount of medication taken, or culture-dependent population norms for psychometric tests, it will not be possible to compare therapies across cultures, or even within ethnic communities in a given geographical area (Kleinman, 1986; Sartorius, 1987).
5. A fifth important parameter is the focus of evaluation. One may view quality of life narrowly in terms of an individual patient, or widely to encompass his immediate family, and then further in concentric circles to take account the broader community (Ware, 1984). In a sense the focus on an individual

patient comes closest to the contemporary medical specialist point of view; the broad community approach is rather akin to traditional public health approaches. Implicit in this distinction is the important observation that small differences affecting many patients may not be of consequence in a patient-orientated study, whereas the same small differences aggregated across a community may be viewed as having great public health significance. In oncology this issue is currently being debated in studies examining the value of prophylactic or 'adjuvant' chemotherapy following primary surgery for breast cancer (Simon, 1987; Cuzick, Steward *et al.*, 1987a,b).

Contemporary Definition of Quality of Life

While no consensus has emerged, it is reasonable to propose some pragmatic definitions of quality of life against which contemporary measures can be assessed and the emerging cohort of trials evaluated. The point of departure for such a definition of quality is the statement of the goals of medical therapy. The intent of medical therapy in this model is to return the patient to a day-to-day functional state no different from that before the onset of the disease. In other words, from a functional point of view the goal is to have day-to-day living unimpeded by either the disease or its treatment. Using such a model, the patient serves as his or her own internal control, thus circumventing concerns about transcultural and intra-cultural norms for quality of life outcome. An important corollary follows. If patients serve as their own internal controls, change in quality of life outcome over time is more important than initial score or specific score at a given time. However, validation studies of this type of tool have confirmed that patient groups stratified for extent of disease and other recognized prognostic parameters have measurably different quality of life scores.

The quality of life construct which emerges from the contemporary literature is function-orientated. As such it seems cross-culturally valid, though confirmatory studies are in their infancy. The construct includes four component parts:

 i. physical and occupational function;
 ii. psychological state;
iii. social interaction;
 iv. somatic sensation.

Physical and occupational function refers to measures of daily activity. Inquiries about the ability to carry on with one's daily activities do not distinguish between housework activities and workforce activities requiring similar effort, concentration and expenditure of energy. In designing such instruments efforts have been made to avoid the 'capping' phenomenon. Many physical and occupational function measures are designed for use in rehabilitation settings with particular focus on dissecting the lower and midrange of functional ability. Thus patients whose function is good are not accurately discriminated from each other by many of these measures (Katz and Arpom, 1976; Schipper *et al.*, 1984).

For the purposes of quality of life studies, psychological state includes issues such as anxiety, depression, anger and fear. As in any test which is designed to provide an overview, there are sacrifices in depth and detail of analysis. Thus the psychological function measures in quality of life tests are brief and may serve to draw attention to major psychological disability but are not in themselves adequate to make a specific diagnosis.

Social interaction reflects the patient's ability to maintain useful social contact with family, friends, and work and community colleagues. It is the cement of community structure. When some early data suggested to our group that social interaction might be the most powerful contributor to quality of life outcome, we were somewhat surprised. We should not have been. Our naivety was best summarized by one correspondent who reminded us that solitary confinement and sensory deprivation have been widely used, powerful tools in the hands of 'correctional' agencies for hundreds of years.

Somatic sensation refers to pain, nausea, vomiting, and other physical sensations which one assumes impinge on a patient's ability to carry on with day-to-day activities. Whereas the first three components of quality of life intuitively and mathematically can be shown to be independent, the emergence of somatic sensation, which would seem to contribute to each of the other factors, as an independent factor may seem somewhat surprising. Most cancer quality of life research groups include measures of nausea and vomiting, hair loss etc. because they reflect the common observable side-effects of anticancer therapy. There are suggestions that the somatic discomfort, identifiably related to treatment, may lead to a quality of outcome different from apparently equivalent discomfort attributed to the disease process itself.

To be useful, a quality of life measure should satisfy the following criteria:

1. It should be disease-specific, that is, the measure should be specific enough to the disease population to detect differences in functional state among patients in a given disease group. In other words, unlike broad-based medical quality of life indices that are designed to measure the medical functional state of free living populations, these tests should take into account that patients have already been diagnosed as having an illness and should concentrate on distinguishing functional states within this population.
2. The index should be functionally orientated, addressing itself to those day-to-day living issues that represent the global construct of functional quality of life.
3. It should be designed for patient self-administration and not require the intervention of interviewers or health professionals for its administration.

4. The questions designed should be of general applicability, ease and consistency of interpretation, and of a number small enough to permit high compliance despite repeated administration.
5. The questionnaire should be designed for repeated use, in order that the patient's score can be followed over a period of time to evaluate trends both within patients and between groups.
6. It should be sensitive across the range of clinical practice, being able to distinguish not only patients who are obviously well from those terminally ill, but more significantly, degrees of dysfunction between patients with varying extent of disease and intensity of therapeutic intervention.
7. The instrument design should have adequately demonstrated face, content, construct and concurrent validity as well as reliability.

Numerous avenues have been followed in the development of quality of life measures. Possibly the earliest quality of life measure was the Karnofsky Performance Index, which was devised forty years ago to provide a physical function representation of the extent of disease (Karnofsky and Burchenal, 1949). For many years the Karnofsky Index and its compressed analogue the Zubrod Scale were the only patient outcome measures incorporated into cancer clinical trials. The tool was designed by physicians, the scores assigned by physicians, and results interpreted by physicians. Many quality of life measures today are likewise strongly physician-orientated (Minet *et al.*, 1987; Evans *et al.*, 1985; Pezim and Nicholls, 1985). Others derived from a nursing and/or psychology point of view may come a little closer to the patient perspective, emphasizing psychological parameters, sexuality, and life satisfaction (Padilla *et al.*, 1983; Schottenfeld and Robbins, 1970). More recently, quality of life measures have been devised having a strong patient orientation, but bringing to bear as well the perspectives of a broad team of health care providers including physicians, nurses, social workers, and clergymen. It is from such measures that the overall construct described above has emerged.

The emergence of practical quality of life indices today has been made possible by three conceptual developments: the recognition that quality of life encompasses more than physical attributes of disease; the emergence of a generalizable construct, a pragmatic function-related definition of quality of life; and the recognition that there are necessary trade-offs between generalizability and disease-specific depth of analysis.

When Karnofsky proposed his scale he did it from the clearly held perspective of a physician as principal determinant of the success of therapy, and his orientation as a monitor of physical function. While at that time there were occasional studies examining psychological and psychiatric attributes of cancer, these did not represent the clinical mainstream. It was generally held that if the disease process were not in check, little else mattered. From the perspective of the time, the Karnofsky scale had great face validity, it seemed logical.

From today's perspective it is easy to be a critic. Yates *et al.*'s (1980) validation study, done more than thirty years later, shows that scores obtained by different professional external observers correlate relatively well, and that low Karnofsky scores are in general predictive of short survival. Further, Karnofsky performance status is now accepted as an independent prognostic factor and is incorporated into the staging of many malignant diseases, particularly lung cancer, and testis cancer (Orr and Aisner, 1986). However, from a psychometric point of view the scale is weak. For example, there are no studies which establish the scalability of the tool. In other words, a deterioration in score from 80 to 60 may bear no relationship to a deterioration from 50 to 30. None the less, the Karnofsky Index served as the first relatively reproducible functional outcome measure used in cancer clinical trials and is today included as a baseline measure in most advanced disease trials.

In 1976 Priestman and Baum conducted a prescient study. They recognized that quality of life was a patient-centred function that encompassed measures of psychological state, functional capacity, social interaction and effectiveness of therapy. Their test consisted of ten simple questions to which a patient was requested to provide an answer as an X on a 10cm line whose ends represented the extremes of good and bad. Though the linear analogue technique had been widely validated in the psychological literature, this represented the first time that this approach had been introduced to a cancer clinical trial. The authors' very brief report provided remarkable clues to the robustness of the functional quality of life concept and its clinical practicality. Patient scores seemed not to be influenced by the presence or absence of the physician at the time the test was taken. The overall quality of life score, which was the simple summation of the numerical values of the ten questions, improved if the patients achieved an objective response to chemotherapy, but remained stable or deteriorated in those patients for whom medical treatment was ineffective. When the test was given on successive days during chemotherapy administration, quality of life scores fell at the beginning of treatment only to level off and improve in the days after chemotherapy was completed. Further, during treatment a four medicine regimen impaired quality of life more than a two medicine regimen. Thus this simple test, almost devoid of rigorous psychometric development, suggested that quality of life was in fact measurable. Patients who were obviously sick had a worse quality of life, which improved as they got better and which could be affected to a greater or lesser extent by the toxicity of treatment.

In 1981 Spitzer *et al.* (1981) brought to bear contemporary psychometric techniques on the issues of scalability and reliability of measures of quality of life. The items selected were drawn from three matched panels each of which included cancer patients, their relatives, those with other chronic diseases and their relatives, healthy persons stratified by age, physicians, nurses, social workers, other health professionals and clergy. A series of data reduction steps ultimately led to two tools. The first, 'The Quality of Life Index' encompassed five items each scored in the integer range of 0–2 and summed. The observations were made by professionals. An observer confidence measure was also included. The second was 'Uniscale'. It was a single item linear analogue scale in which the observer was asked to mark with an X 'the appropriate place within the bar to indicate your rating of this person's quality of life during the past week'. Parallel self-administered questionnaires were developed for both the Quality of Life scale and Uniscale. The overall correlations between physician-observer and patient self-administered scores were poor. They did not exceed 0.63. In general interobserver correlations were better for sicker patients. The most seriously ill patients were unable to complete the questionnaire. Inasmuch as this study was a calibrational trial, the Spitzer Index was not extensively compared with lengthy or more elaborate measures of physical and occupational function, psychological state and social interaction in order to provide evidence of concurrent validity. The study attracted considerable attention and the index was incorporated into a number of clinical trials. Possibly the most provocative was the National Hospice Study (NHS) which was intended to provide objective and hopefully supportive measures of the efficacy of the burgeoning hospice movement (Morris *et al*., 1986). Unfortunately neither Uniscale nor the five-item tool was particularly discriminatory. In retrospect this might have been predicted from the relatively poor correlations observed in the calibration study. None the less Spitzer's work represented a watershed. It demonstrated that it was possible to develop quality of life indices, and that it was feasible to administer and score them.

It remained for the next generation of investigators to bring to bear fully test instrument validation and development procedures. Throughout this period one senses in the literature a twofold intellectual struggle. The pragmatics of quality of life assessment demand that a test be repeatable over time, yet the more frequently one wishes to repeat the test the greater the necessity of brevity. However, brevity comprises both the sensitivity of the tool and its ability to discriminate degrees of debility. The second debate is between the psychometricians and the clinicians. The psychometrician has developed a mathematically rigorous, and in the eyes of some, seemingly endless series of scientific tests of validity and reliability. He is unhappy unless a large number of these criteria are met. The clinician wishes to define the clinical limits of a tool, and within these limits use it and interpret it. To this extent the painstaking psychometric work of the European Organization for Research and Treatment of Cancer (EORTC) Psychological Group (Aaronson and Beckmann, 1987) can be contrasted with the more global approaches of Padilla *et al*. (1983), Gough *et al*. (1983), Selby *et al*. (1984), and our group (Schipper *et al*., (1984). Each of these clinician groups have developed scales having considerable psychometric validity. Factor analysis, concurrent validation studies, measures of internal consistency, tests of interobserver reliability and even measures of social desirability, which attempts to quantitate the extent to which a patient seeks to please his physician with his answer, have all been included in the instrument development process.

Possibly the Functional Living Index for Cancer (FLIC) is the most widely used current instrument (Schipper *et al.*, 1984). It is employed by most of the American clinical trials groups, and shares with the EORTC scales a role as the basis of a World Health Organization scale which is in the late stages of development. These scales are not etched in stone. Possibly the World Health Organization scale will be widely enough adopted so as to provide a global basis of comparison for clinical trials outcomes. If one is to anticipate the nature of quality of life measures in a particular clinical trial, it is likely that there will be a core quality of life measure consisting of between twenty and thirty questions that can be easily repeated at intervals as short as every two weeks. In addition, specific disease-related items might be added as modules in order further to explicate differences in overall quality of life outcome which might be anticipated to emerge. Thus issues of respiratory function which might offer little insight in a myeloma trial, may be of great significance in a lung cancer study.

The study of quality of life measurement has advanced far enough that in designing and reviewing trials, as an essential minimum, even the most pragmatic clinician should demand that his tools have adequate face validity, construct validity concurrent validity, inter-rater reliability, and internal consistency (Schipper and Levitt, 1985).

A number of trials have been completed which illustrate the potential of quality of life studies in cancer therapy. Though their trial was completed before the emergence of the briefer quality of life tools, Sugarbaker and his colleagues (1982) were able to demonstrate that what at first appeared to be an obvious treatment in aid of quality of life, was, when appropriately studied, just the contrary. With informed consent, patients with extremity sarcomas were randomized to either amputation and chemotherapy, or limb-sparing surgery plus radiation and chemotherapy. The declared a priori prediction was that those patients whose limbs were spared would have an improved quality of life without an increased mortality. In fact those whose limbs were spared had an impaired quality of life as interpreted in this trial, manifest mostly through a functional degradation in sexual relationships. This study is an interesting example of how a single dysfunctional area may materially affect overall quality of life. As such it raises the issue of whether quality of life is in fact a uniform whole which can be represented as a single item or whether it is best represented as a family of scores for physical and occupational function, psychological state, social interaction, and somatic sensation. It is a moot point whether the significant sexual dysfunction found in Sugarbaker's study could have been detected by a single-item test such as Uniscale, by intermediate range tests such as the FLIC, or only by highly detailed interrogations using batteries of tests administered at long intervals. However, it serves to point out clearly the balance the investigator must strike between breadth and ease on one hand, and depth and complexity on the other.

The medical literature is rife with studies using 'quality of life' as a buzz word. Appendix A provides a tabular overview of some of these studies. It illustrates the diversity of approaches, and the conceptual and procedural deficiencies associated with this emerging field of study. To their credit they reflect a concern for more than the physical attributes of disease, and possibly more than survival and disease-free survival as well. Some infer a quality of life benefit from surgical procedures which are less disfiguring. Yet there is evidence in the recent mastectomy literature in particular that after a short interval, for many patients, traditional mastectomy offers no disadvantage in quality of life as compared to lesser surgical procedures, possibly because of alleviation of fear about recurrence, and concern about bearing a diseased breast. If one accepts the definition of quality of life upon which this current argument is based, then studies which deal with the narrow specifics of improved comfort for a given surgical appliance, or relative amounts of nausea and vomiting, cannot be called quality of life studies. It may be that these manoeuvres do influence quality of life, but this can only be determined by asking as well more global quality of life questions. In other words, in the quality-of-life-plus-module model, to analyse only the module is inadequate.

Design of the Quality of Life Clinical Trial

With reasonably mature quality of life tools in hand it has become apparent that specific techniques for conducting and analysing a quality of life trial are necessary. Quality of life is a labile parameter, and unlike the curves which emerge from survival and disease-free survival studies, these data are not in general representable by monotonically decreasing curves. Further, since the patient serves as his own internal control in many of these studies, timing issues are critical. In a survival or disease-free survival trial, a patient lost to follow-up for ten years and then recovered and found to be alive and free from disease is, from a statistical point of view, as valid a survivor as someone who had been observed at monthly intervals for the duration. This is not true for quality of life studies. Thus issues of physician and patient compliance, and accrual and follow-up are critical to the statistical and clinical validity of any study. The guidelines which follow serve to offer consistency in this endeavour.

There are three situations in which quality of life as an outcome measure is likely to be useful: two of these relate to the question of 'does the end justify the means?'. The first is when there is justification for a no treatment arm because no known treatment has any influence on survival and all have some degree of toxicity. The second is when marked improvements in survival over the conventional therapy are anticipated at the expense of increased acute or long-term toxicity. The third situation is one in which some new method of ameliorating the side-effects of treatment is being tested and not the anticancer treatment itself. These are all situations in which a quality of life treatment effect is anticipated and all are appropriate to evaluation by a Phase III trial rather than a Phase I or II trial.

Consent to enter a patient into a clinical trial must necessarily be sought after a diagnosis of cancer has been made and consequently no pre-diagnosis or pre-cancer quality of life baseline can be determined. The first assessment serves as a baseline for the individual patient against which all subsequent values will be compared. There is no question but that the diagnosis itself will influence some of the components of the measure because of the patient's anxiety regarding the course, treatment and eventual outcome of the disease. Naturally the amount of information patients receive prior to completion of the first questionnaire will influence their response and this must therefore be standardized. Since the effect of treatment is to be evaluated, the first quality of life assessment should take place before initial treatment and at a consistent time in relation to that treatment for all patients.

Unlike survival, quality of life is a measure which may be repeated several times thus providing a picture of the course of a disease and its treatment. Obviously there will be fluctuations in overall score and component scores both as a result of debility due to disease and treatment, and as a result of intercurrent life events. Testing must be frequent enough to detect important fluctuations but not so frequent that patients become irritated or fatigued by questionnaire completion, or tend to remember their previous response. Currently used measures of quality of life are repeated at intervals of one week to three months. Careful consideration of the treatment protocol and the purpose of using quality of life as an outcome measure should enable determination of an appropriate testing interval (Figure 2). Differences in the treatment protocol between groups are not necessarily a problem as long as the testing intervals are the same. However, when toxic episodes result in treatment delays for specific patients, this will tend to obscure the quality of life profile over time for a given treatment and may therefore result in less well-defined treatment differences. Measurements made close to toxic events register temporary fluctuations and those that are made distant from these events assess overall trends.

Duration of follow-up is an important consideration when using quality of life measurements to assess treatment differences in clinical trials. When disease-free interval and/or survival is anticipated to be short, then follow-up should continue until death. Often patients become too debilitated to complete questionnaires at which point quality of life follow-up must cease. In cases where patients show no evidence of disease after an initial treatment period, follow-up should continue in order to assess any long-term effects which outlast the treatment period. At this point the frequency of testing could be reduced. Very different conclusions may be drawn depending upon whether the follow-up period is long enough to detect long-term effects of treatment (Figure 3).

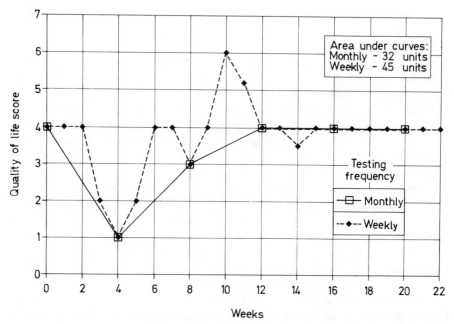

Figure 2. The importance of frequency of testing is illustrated here. Assuming the 'true' quality of life is represented by the broken line, measuring at weekly intervals or at monthly intervals leads to 'significantly' different profiles. Note also that data missed cannot be recaptured

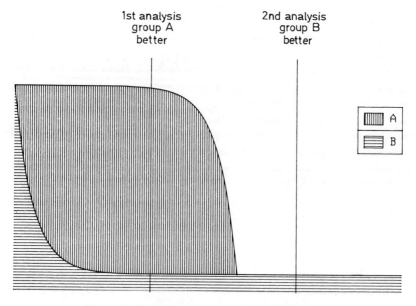

Figure 3. The influence of duration of follow-up

Analysis of the Quality of Life Parameter

The usual analytical methods associated with Phase III clinical trials are not necessarily appropriate for the analysis of quality of life data. Survival or disease-free survival are customarily represented by logarithmic plots of the cumulative proportion of patients surviving through each time period, starting at diagnosis. This method deals only with two points in time—diagnosis, and death or recurrence of disease—and completely ignores what happens to the patient in between. It has been suggested that quality of life could be analysed in the same fashion using some specified low value as an endpoint (Fayers and Jones, 1983). Aside from the inevitable but unfortunate connotation that life is no longer worth living once this value is reached, such a method completely ignores the purpose of using quality of life as an outcome measure. It is the description of the fluctuations in a patient's overall well-being from diagnosis to death, in other words the effects of the process of the disease and its treatment, which are relevant to the quality of life measure. Also the survival analysis has a negative focus and ignores the possibility of improvement.

When a set of measurements is obtained at regular time intervals and events which may influence the value of these measurements occur, then a common method of assessing their effect is to perform an interrupted time series analysis. This method takes into account random and cyclical fluctuations in the measure when testing for the statistical significance of the effects of events and interventions. The technique is applicable to a single time series representing an individual or a group as well as to the comparison of two separate groups. However, since the statistical model required to analyse the differences between two or more groups is more complicated, computer programs for group comparisons are not generally available. Until these programs become available, time series analysis will not be a useful method for Phase III trials.

If measurements are taken at regular intervals on all patients, then analysis of variance (ANOVA) procedures can be used to describe trends over time and to test for differences in these trends between treatment arms of a trial (Kirk, 1968). Figure 4 illustrates one possible configuration of results for two groups of patients over several measurement periods. Several questions can be asked of such data in the form of statistical significance tests: (i) is there an overall trend in the quality of life measures over time, combining data from both groups; (ii) is there a difference in the overall quality of life for the two groups averaged over all time periods; (iii) is there a difference in the trend over time for the two treatments.

A trend in the data is described in the ANOVA by breaking it down into its various components. One could choose to test for linear trend by drawing a straight line through the points but this may not be a sufficient description of the data. The linear trend may be subtracted from the overall trend and tests for quadratic and/or higher order trends can be performed (this is limited by the number of measurements made and the order of the highest trend which can be tested is one less than the number of measurements). A quadratic trend describes a curve with one inflection point, a cubic trend describes a curve with two inflection points, etc.

In the example shown in Figure 4 there is no overall difference between the treatment groups when the data are averaged over all time periods for each group. There is a distinct trend over time which may be broken down into six possible components averaged over treatment groups because there are seven measurements for each individual. 'Eyeballing' the data would indicate the possibility of both a linear and a cubic trend component both of which are statistically significant. However, there is no quadratic trend. Neither is there any residual difference over time not accounted for by the linear and cubic trends.

Quite clearly the trends in the two treatment groups are not the same and tests for differences in trend bear this out. A test for difference in linear trend

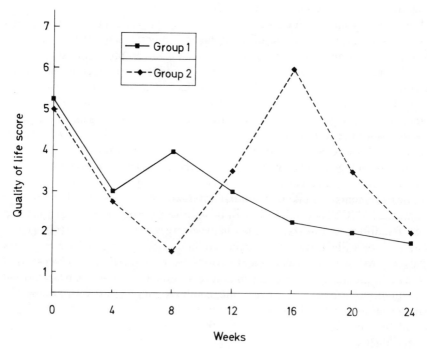

Figure 4. Mean Quality of Life scores at four-week intervals for treatment arms receiving minimal therapy (Group 1) and more agressive therapy (Group 2) for the same disease. Hypothetical data were constructed for four patients in each group and an ANOVA was performed. Results of the analysis are discussed in the test

indicates that if a separate linear regression line were drawn through the data from each group, the two lines would not have the same slope. Since the two lines are obviously very different in the magnitude of their two inflections, a significant difference in cubic trend might be expected and is present. Not surprisingly there is no difference in quadratic trend.

In this example Group 1 might represent patients who received minimal therapy between their diagnosis at time zero and six weeks later. Treatment plus the disease process led to a deterioration in their quality of life but after treatment was concluded a brief recovery occurred followed by a progressive decline. In contrast Group 2 might represent patients who received a far more aggressive therapy which led to both a more dramatic deterioration and a more dramatic subsequent improvement. Since the final result at week 24 was very little different in the two groups, the question of which therapy is preferable is hard to answer. However the extent to which Group 2's data fall below those of Group 1 is less than the extent to which they subsequently exceed Group 1's data. Therefore one might argue that the treatment received by Group 2 was superior.

This type of ANOVA, known as a repeated measures ANOVA, requires rather restrictive statistical assumptions which may not be met by the data. In addition to the standard ANOVA assumptions of normality, random sampling, equality of variance across treatment groups and independence of the numerator and denominator of the F-ratio, the repeated measures ANOVA requires that the covariances between each pair of measurements on the same individuals should be equal. This latter requirement is often not met but procedures are available for dealing with the problem, that is, by using an approximate F-test.

An alternative, less restrictive analysis is a multivariate analysis of variance which performs a simultaneous analysis on all measurements for an individual at the same time. Exactly the same hypotheses may be tested as with the repeated measures ANOVA but there is an additional advantage that the components of the quality of life measure could also be analysed simultaneously, and their relative contribution to group differences at various points in time could be assessed (Morrison, 1974; Finn, 1978).

A difficulty with these and most other forms of analysis of multiple measurement data is that methods of dealing with missing information are problematic. In the case of the repeated measures ANOVA, computer programs can analyse data with missing observations but often they give the wrong estimates (SAS Institute Inc., 1985). It is, however, possible to correct the output using techniques developed by Milliken and Johnson (1985) but they are complicated and time-consuming. In the case of the multivariate ANOVA, the computer programs delete a whole set of data if any observations in the series are missing because mathematically the analysis is not possible in this circumstance.

An even more serious analytic problem results from patient deaths at different times during the trial. Missing data in a series can be adjusted for appropriately during analysis but there is no way of dealing with the absence of information after a patient dies. The consequence is that comparative analysis of group data can only be performed prior to death of the first patient. Repeat analysis could be conducted on the successively smaller remaining group of patients but it would be necessary to make an adjustment in required significance levels to allow for the reanalysis of data. Alternatively, data from subgroups of patients who die within specified time periods could be analysed separately. This emphasizes the need to use homogeneous groups of patients in a comparative trial or to plan for subgroup analysis when calculating the required sample size. A corollary of the problem of missing data is the importance of patient follow-up by research staff. Quality of life studies require more data handling resources than equivalent studies which measure response and survival. There are more data points per encounter, and the non-recoverability of data makes an efficient patient teaching and prompting mechanism essential. Assuming a biweekly testing schedule, one data manager can be expected to handle not more than 50 patients, including patient accrual, prompting and follow-up, and basic data entry.

We have defined quality of life as a composite of four factors: physical and occupational function, psychological state, social interactions and somatic sensation. Do the studies we undertake lead to a single composite score, four individual component scores or both?

The individual component scores cannot be considered definitive evaluators of psychological or social functions. They can draw attention to major areas of dysfunction, leading to more detailed examination. To date, no quality of life measure has been constructed in which the relative weightings of each component factor have been clinically determined, a priori. The factor-analysis-based instrument design employed to date assumes each question contributes equally to the overall score. The weighting of each factor in that score is thus a function of the number of questions asked. Thus an overall quality of life score measures quality of life as empirically defined by the particular test structure, but provides little insight into the contribution each factor makes to the total outcome.

At present, the optimal approach is to provide both overall quality of life scores plus the contributory component scores. This provides an overall assessment while affording insight into the mechanisms underlying the outcome. It is entirely possible using such an approach to imagine a clinical trial where overall quality of life outcomes are similar, but in which an examination of the outcome factor by factor reveals trade-offs, such as improved occupational function at the expense of social interaction. Offering this dual analysis circumvents the difficult factor-weighting issues, while providing insights into underlying mechanisms. Such an approach does not require increased patient numbers.

Quality of Life Trials: Interpretation

How does one interpret a quality of life trial? A quality of life result is distinct from but complementary to a survival or disease-free survival result. It does not seem likely that we will in the foreseeable future be able to construct a unifying hypothesis, analogous to what Einstein sought for physics, linking survival quality with survival quantity. At any point in the clinical spectrum there will be trade-offs to make. At the present time we are able to discuss among medical specialists and scientists disease-free survival and survival differences between various therapies. We have quantitative data on which to base trials to extend survival. As quality of life trials emerge we will for the first time have broadly acceptable data upon which to look at overall human function in the context of treatment for malignant disease. Recall that this is functionally defined quality of life. It is for the most part not quality of life measured against some absolute external standard, but as measured against a patient's past experience and expectation. That is a limitation of the quality of life model as it currently exists. Such a model does not work well in the context of medicine as a tool to improve society as a whole, because in our construction it is not possible numerically to elaborate total achievement. In contrast these issues do not even arise in a survival or disease-free survival study, because the endpoint is relapse or death which are unequivocal. So we are faced with trade-offs. The trade-off is finite time to death or relapse against non-linear and potentially infinite improvements in quality of life.

In a trial measuring both survival (or disease-free survival) and quality of life, there are three possible trial outcomes. The first outcome is that when measured over the pre-defined time interval of the trial, therapy A is superior to B for both survival and quality of life (Figure 5). Choose therapy A as the baseline for the next study. What is more difficult, however, is to decide whether the next trial seeks primarily to improve quality of life, possibly by decreasing the toxicity of treatment A, or to provide additional survival by adding to the toxicity of A. We have two parameters to balance. To some extent the state of chemotherapy for advanced non-seminomatous carcinomas of the testis represents this clinical conundrum. We are curing 80 per cent of patients. The treatment is of relatively short duration and while the toxicities during treatment are difficult, the long-term morbidity, though not overwhelming, is considerably greater than we initially anticipated. In this setting quality of life data provide added impetus to the need to identify subgroups of high-risk patients who might benefit from more aggressive therapies.

The next level of complexity is the clinical trial in which the survival of A is better than survival of B but quality of life in A and B are equal, or quality of life in A is better than B but survival of A and B are equal (Figure 6). Choose the better arm. However, the next trial choice is defined in a different way than was the case when we were restricted to survival and disease-free survival

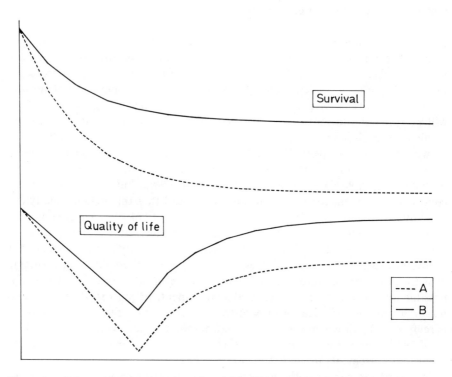

Figure 5.   Schematic representation of a trial in which one arm is, at all points, superior
to the other both for survival and quality of life

data. Now one must dissect either biologically or functionally the mechanisms underlying the inferior arm, and seek to manipulate it while not compromising the superior arm. As an example, it may be that two years of Melphelan and 5-Fluorouracil are therapeutically equivalent to one year of Cyclophosphamide Methotrexate and 5-Fluorouracil in preventing recurrences in stage II breast cancer. The per treatment toxicity of Melphelan 5FU is probably less than that of CMF. Do you shorten the therapy with Melphelan 5FU?

The third possible outcome is the most difficult. In this situation survival outcome of A is superior to that of B, but quality of life outcome of B is superior to that achieved with A (Figure 7). Without a biomedical equivalent of the Unified Field Theory there is no clear answer to this 'Paradoxical Trial'. However, there is a choice. For an individual patient there is a trade-off in which, for the first time, he can be a reasonably informed participant with his physician. For the trials designer there are two equally ethical approaches. One may seek either to alleviate the quality of life disadvantage of the survival superior trial, or attempt to improve survival without unduly compromising quality of life in the functional-outcome superior arm. At a given time in the evolution of

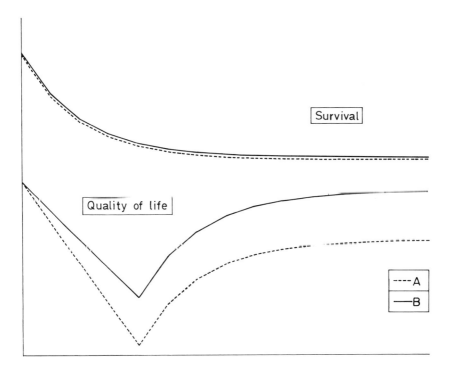

Figure 6.   A trial comparing two therapies offering equal survival but different quality of life outcomes

treatment of a particular cancer the potential therapeutic gain from a survival-orientated trial may be less than that of a quality of life orientated trial. One must take that into account. One can predict some heated debates in clinical trials group steering committees. However, these debates will be based on data for quality of life which are in their own context as sound as the survival and disease-free survival data to which we are considerably more accustomed.

Quality of life as a concept is a powerful tool. As currently defined, it is the common final destination of all interventions in aid of our sick patient. If as physicians and health planners we embrace the concept, we find ourselves speaking from common ground with our patients. More traditional biometric measures notwithstanding, we are able to speak in terms our patients understand, and to speak in a language that can be seen to represent society's goals. When physicians restrict themselves to talking about PO2, creatinine clearance, tumour size and survival, we are at a distance from the population and are always vulnerable to the societal 'so what'. Now we seem to have been able to bring medical science to the deepest recesses of individual liberty. The potential for abuse is great. Consider the following examples:

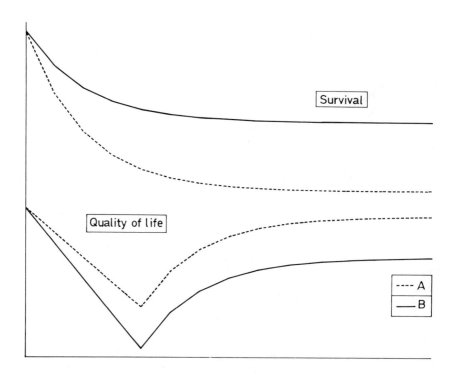

Figure 7.   The difficult outcome: The Paradoxical Trial. The complexity of
interpretation is increased if the relative outcomes reverse over time

1. Two treatments, neither of them curative, are compared. There are a few
   unexpected long-term survivors of a treatment which is expensive and whose
   quality of life cost is great. A treatment which cures none but prolongs life
   for many carries with it a relatively good quality of life until death. Further,
   the treatment is inexpensive. We must not in the name of economics cease all
   investigation into the more expensive treatment. The fact that a few patients
   are cured where none had been cured before provides a biological clue that
   cannot be ignored. Patients must be informed of the high risks of the occasionally curative therapy. The community may wish to focus its resources in
   an attempt to exploit the biological pathway by restricting such investigational treatments to a small number of centres. However, these data should
   not provide an econometrically based excuse for halting biological investigation. After all, one can materially but temporarily improve the quality of
   life of Hodgkin's patients with morphine, while this curable disease takes its
   relentless and fatal course in the absence of established therapy.

2. A corollary occurs when comparing treatment for different diseases. If the treatment for disease X is better from a quality of life point of view than the treatment for disease Y, one might be tempted to focus resources on treatment X. Dollar for dollar, given the current state of the art, there is more to be gained by treating a population of patients with disease X than those with disease Y. If you stop treating disease Y, in the short term you save money. In the long term you freeze medicine in its tracks. One must carefully balance resources so as to find out why treatment Y is inferior and seek to develop new treatments for the disease.
3. The emergence of the quality of life construct makes treatment of individual patients a matter of trade-offs as well. Quality of life is not an outcome measure superior to traditional biological response. It is a patient-centred end measure which is complementary. We have come to accept that there are limitations to the strictly biological approach to medicine. There will be a temptation to recommend to a patient the treatment which offers the best quality of life. That is as narrowly limiting as current survival-orientated management. We must as physicians become accustomed to incorporating both parts of the model into our judgements and to communicating them to our patients, so that to the extent they wish to be partners in therapeutic decision-making, they have the facts.
4. If one is not careful in using the quality of life concept, one can fall into the trap of therapeutic nihilism. Some studies of the translocation of adjuvant chemotherapy for breast cancer from investigational trials groups centred in university-based hospitals to the community, suggest that the established benefits of adjuvant chemotherapy are being compromised in the community by an ill-advised focus on quality of life. Patients are being given less drug because physicians do not want to make them sick. The work of Hryniuk and Levine (1986) and others suggests that dose intensity in this setting is important. Further there is evidence that the side-effects of chemotherapy may have a less adverse effect on a patient's quality of life than similar side-effects attributable to the disease. In the face of these data, backing off from treatment for fear of toxicity, without having in hand carefully designed quality of life studies with adequate follow-up periods, is ill-advised and ethically questionable.

The growth of the clinical trial in cancer research has been driven by a great social need to control a dreaded disease, and by the existence of technologies and approaches which offer the promise of solution. Our understanding of the biological basis of cellular control forms the essence of therapeutic approaches to control a family of diseases whose essential feature is a breakdown in cellular growth regulation. When it became apparent that we could alter, if only transiently, the natural history of some cancers, we began a series of clinical, biologically based trials to confirm these results. It took almost two decades to evolve a methodology which defines adequately tumour response, disease-free survival and survival. While anecdotal reports are not to be dismissed out of hand for the observations they may offer, trials which do not adhere to rigorous guidelines should be viewed with suspicion because they may be either uninterpretable, or unsuitable for comparison to other similar trials, or both.

Quality of life is a relatively new and still evolving outcome concept. To a certain extent it is popular ahead of its time, making it vulnerable to both abuse and discredit, particularly through oversimplification. The outcome measures which are now available are good second-generation approximations, and the guidelines which have evolved for their use make possible reasonable interpretations of clinical trial results. It is appropriate to expect quality of life as an outcome measure to be incorporated into Phase III clinical trials now and in the future. We should, however, expect to apply these outcome measures in conjunction with more traditional measures such as survival and disease-free survival. This increasing sophistication in trial analysis only parallels the increasing sophistication and understanding of the malignant process.

References

Aaronson, N.K. and Beckmann, J. (eds) (1987). *The Quality of Life of Cancer Patients*, New York: Raven.

Arora, R., Sager, J. and Butler, R. (1986). *Cardiology Clinics*, **4** (2), 305–12.

Bell, D.R., Tannock, I.F. and Boyd, N.F. (1985). *British Journal of Medicine*, **51**, 577–80.

Bergner, M., Bobbitt, R.A., Pollard, W.E., Martin, D.P. and Gilson, B.S. (1976). *Medical Care*, **XIV** (1), 57–67.

Brinkley, D. (1985). *British Medical Journal*, **291** (6497), 685.

Brown, G.W. (1987). *British Medical Journal*, **294**, 1026–8.

Calman, K.C. (1984). *Journal of Medical Ethics*, **10**, 124–7.

Canellos, G.P. (1973). *Seminar Hematology*, **20**, 1.

Carter, S.K. and Selaway, O. (1977). *National Cancer Institute Monograph*, **45**, 81–92.

Carter, S.K., Selaway, O. and Slavik, M. (1977). *National Cancer Institute Monograph*, **45**, 75–80.

Cohen, J. (1977). *Statistical Power Analysis for the Behavioural Sciences*, New York: Academic Press.

Cribb, A. (1985). *Journal of Medical Ethics*, **11**, 142–5.

Croog, S.H., Levine, S., Testa, M., Brown, B., Bulpitt, C.J., Jenkins, C.D., Klerman, G.L. and Williams, G.H. (1986). *New England Journal of Medicine*, **314**, 1657–64.

Cuzick, J., Stewart, H., Peto, R., Fisher, B., Kaae, S., Johansen, H., Lythgoe, J.P. and Prescott, R.J. (1987a). *Cancer Treatment Reports*, **71**, 7–11.

Cuzick, J., Stewart, H., Peto, R., Baum, M., Fisher, B., Host, H., Lythgoe, J.P., Ribeiro, G., Scheurlen, H. and Wallgren, A. (1987b). *Cancer Treatment Reports*, **71**, 15–25.

De Haes, J.C.J.M. and Van Knippenberg, F.C.E. (1985). *Social Science Medicine*, **20**, 809–17.

De Haes, J.C.J.M. and Welvaart, K. (1985). *Journal of Surgical Oncology*, **28**, 123–5.
Edlund, M. and Tancredi, L. (1985). *Perspectives in Biology and Medicine*, **28**, 591–608.
Evans, A.E., Gilbert, E.S. and Zandstra, R. (1970). *Cancer*, **26**, 404.
Evans, R. and Manninen, D. (1985). *New England Journal of Medicine*, **312** (24), 1579–80.
Evans, R., Manninen, D., Garrison, L., Hart, L.G., Blagg, C., Gutman, R., Hull, A. and Lowrie, E.G. (1985). *New England Journal of Medicine*, **312** (9), 553–9.
Eriksson, B., Oberg, K., Alm, G., Karlsson, A., Lundqvist, G., Magnusson, A., Wide, L. and Wilander, E. (1987). *Cancer Treatment Reports*, **7**, 31–7.
Farber, S., Diamond, L.K., Mercer, R.D., Sylvester, R.F. and Wolfe, J.A. (1948). *New England Journal of Medicine*, **238**, 787.
Fayers, P.M. and Jones, D.R. (1983). *Statistics in Medicine*, **2**, 429–46.
Ferrans, C. and Powers, M. (1985). *Advances in Nursing Science*, **8** (1), 15–24.
Finn, J.D. (1978). *Multivariance: Univariate and Multivariate analyses of variance, covariance, regression and repeated measures*, Users Guide, Version VI, Release 2.
Flanagan, J.C. (1982). *Archives of Physical Medicine and Rehabilitation*, **63**, 56–9.
Garnick, M.B. (1985). *Journal of Clinical Oncology*, **3**, 294
Gehan, E.A. (1961). *Journal of Chronic Diseases*, **13**, 346–53.
Gough, I.R., Furnival, G.M., Schilder, L. and Grove, W. (1983). *European Journal of Cancer and Clinical Oncology*, **19**, 1161–5.
Guyatt, G., Bombardier, C. and Tugwell, P. (1986). *Canadian Medical Association Journal*, **134**, 889–95.
Harrison, P. (1986). *Canadian Medical Association Journal*, **135**, 1294–6.
Henderson, E.S. (1967). *Cancer Research*, **27**, 2570.
Homan, E.R. (1972). *Cancer Chemotherapy Reports*, **3**, 13–19.
Hryniuk, W. and Levine, M.N. (1986). *Journal of Clinical Oncology*, **4**, 1162–70.
Hunt, S., McKenna, S.P., McEwen, J., Backett, E.M., Williams, J. and Papp, E. (1980). *Journal of Epidemiology and Community Health*, **34**, 281–6.
Hunter, Carrie P., Frelick, Robert W., Feldman, Allen R., Bavier, Anne R., Dunlap, Wilma H., Ford, Leslie, Henson, Donald, MacFarlene, Dorothy, Smart, Charles R., Yancik, Rosemary and Yates, Jerome W (1987). *Cancer Treat Rep*, **71**, 559–65.
Karnofsky, D.A. and Burchenal, J.H. (1949). The clinical evaluation of chemotherapeutic agents in cancer. In *Evaluation of Chemotherapeutic Agents*, ed. Mcleod, C.M., New York: Columbia.
Katz, S. and Arpom, C.A. (1976). *International Journal of Health Service*, **6**, 493–508.
Kirk, R.E. (1968). *Experimental Design: Procedures for the Behavioural Sciences*, Belmont, California: Brooks/Cole Publishing Company.
Kleinman, A. (1986). Culture, the quality of life and cancer pain: anthropological and cross-cultural issues. In *Assessment of Quality of Life and Cancer Treatment*, ed. Ventafridda, V. *et al.*, Amsterdam: Excerpt Medical Medica.
Kottke, F.J. (1982). *Archives of Physical Medicine and Rehabilitation*, **63**, 60–2.
Krupinski, J. (1980). *Social Science and Medicine*, **14A**, 203–11.
Kutner, N. (1985). *New England Journal of Medicine*, **312** (24), 1579.
Landesman, S. (1986). *Mental Retardation*, **91**, 14–15.
Medical Research Council Report (1973). *British Medical Journal*, **2**, 381–94.
Milliken, G.A. and Johnson, D.E. (1984). *The Analysis of Messy Data*, Vol. 1: Designed Experiments, Belmont, California: Lifetime Learning Publications.
Milstein, J.M., Cohen, M.E. and Sinks, L.F. (1985). *Cancer*, **56**, 1834–6.
Minet, P., Bartsch, P., Chevalier, Ph., Raets, D., Gras, A., Dejardin-Closon, MTh., Lennes, G. and Leige Lung Group (1987). *Radiotherapy and Oncology*, **8**, 217–30.

Morris, J., Suissa, S., Sherwood, S., Wright, M. and Geer, D. (1986). *Journal of Chronic Diseases*, **39** (1), 47–62.

Morrison, D.F. (1977). *Multivariate Statistical Methods*, 2, New York: McGraw-Hill.

Morton, R.P., Davies, A.D.M., Baker, J., Baker, G.A. and Stell, P.M. (1984). *Clinical Otolaryngol*, **9**, 181–5.

Oakley, C. (1987). *Quarterly Journal of Medicine, New Series*, **62** (239), 181–2.

Orr, S.T. and Aisner, J. (1986). *Cancer Treatment Reports*, **70**, 1423–9.

Padilla, G.V., Presant, C., Grant, M.M., Mether, G., Baer, C. and Finnie (1983). *Research in Nursing & Health*, **6**, 117–26.

Pearlman, R. and Jonsen, A. (1985). *Journal of American Geriatrics Society*, **33**, 334–52.

Pezim, M.E. and Nicholls, R.J. (1985). *British Journal of Surgery*, **72** (1), 31–3.

Presant, C. (1984). *American Journal of Clinical Oncology*, **7**, 571–3.

Priestman, T.J. and Baum, M. (1976). *Lancet*, April, 899–900.

Rozenbaum, E.A., Pliskin, J.S., Barnoon, S. and Chaimovitz, C. (1985). *Israel Journal of Medical Sciences*, **21**, 335–9.

Sartorius, W. (1987). Cross-cultural comparisons of data about quality of life: A sample of issues. In *The Quality of Life of Cancer Patients*, ed. Aaronson, N.K. and Bechman, J., New York: Raven.

SAS Institute (1985). *SAS Users Guide: Statistics Version 5 Edition*, Cary, North Carolina: SAS Institute.

Schipper, H. (1983). *Canadian Medical Association Journal*, **128**, 1367–9.

Schipper, H., Clinch, J., McMurray, A. and Levitt, M. (1984). *Journal of Clinical Oncology*, **2**, 472–83.

Schipper, H. and Levitt, M. (1985). *Cancer Treatment Reports*, **69**, 1115–23.

Schottenfeld, D. and Robbins, G.F. (1970). *Cancer*, **26**, 650–5.

Selby, P. (1985). *British Journal of Hospital Medicine*, May, 266–71.

Selby, P.J., Chapman, J.A.W., Etazade-Amoli, Dalley, D. and Boyd, D.F. (1984). *British Journal of Cancer*, **50**, 13–22.

Slayton, R.E. (1984). *Seminars in Oncology*, **1**, 299.

Spitzer, W.O., Dobson, A. J., Chesterman, E., Levi, J., Shepherd, R., Battista, R.N. and Catchlove, B.R. (1981). *Journal of Chronic Disease*, **34**, 585–97.

Sugarbaker, P.H., Barofsky, I., Rosenberg, S.A. and Granola, F.J. (1982). *Surgery*, **91**, 17–23.

Sugimachi, K., Maekawa, S., Koga, Y., Ueo, H. and Inokuchi, K. (1985). *Surgery, Gynecology & Obstetrics*, **162**, 544–6.

Thomasma, D. (1986). *Clinics in Geriatric Medicine*, **2** (1), 17–27.

Ware, J.E. (1984). *Cancer*, **53**, 2316–26.

Warr, D., McKinney, S. and Tannock, I. (1985). *Journal of Clinical Oncology*, **2**, 1040–6.

Wiklund, I., Lindvall, K. and Swedberg, K. (1986). *Acta Med. Scand*, **220**, 1–3.

Wortman, C.B. and Dunkel-Schietter, C. (1979). *Journal Soc. Issues*, **35**, 120–55.

Wortman, P. and Yeaton, W. (1985). *Controlled Clinical Trials*, **6**, 289–305.

Yates, J.W., Chalmer, B. and McKegney, F.P. (1980). *Cancer*, **45**, 2220–4.

Appendix A: A Tabular Overview of Quality of Life Studies

This table summarizes 37 selected quality of life studies. An x indicates that the specific feature is included in the study. Where the item is blank, the feature is either not considered or not reported.

Section A defines the study population characteristics and the presence of a control group.

Section B groups the quality of life characteristics according to the present definition. In many instances we have had to extrapolate the category from the study report.

Section C reports critical procedural issues related to the conduct of the trial.

P/O: O indicates an external observer as data source, P indicates patient self-assessment.

The lack of definition of quality of life and procedural vagueness in compiling studies is readily apparent.

The authors are indebted to Valerie Powell SRN for her efforts in completing this table.

(NB: the tabulated material begins overleaf.)

	Morris *et al.* (1986)	Ferrans and Powers 1985	Presant (1984)	Oakley (1987)	Landesman (1986)
A. Subject/Controls					
N	1121 + 114	125	130		
Age				Men under 65	Mentally retarded
Disease	Terminal hospice CA inpatients	Dialysis pts 37 grad students 88	Cancer patients	After angioplasty	
Controls	x		x		
B. Content					
Physical:					
overall	x	x		x	
mobility	x	x			
ADL self care	x	x	x		
domestic	x	x	x		
financial		x	x		
occupational	x	x	x	x	
Psychological:					
overall	x	x	x	x	x
depression	x	x		x	
anxiety	x			x	
anger	x				
Social Interaction:					
overall	x	x	x	x	x
recreation			x		
effect on other	x	x			
sexual activity				x	
interest			x	x	

Somatic:			
overall			
nausea			
pain	x	x	
GI	x	x	
sleep		x	
dyspnoea		x	
		x	angina
C. Procedures			
Source P/O	0		P+O
Questionnaire S/O	0		
Named QL	8 measures	Q/L Index	
Validity		x	
Reliability		x	
D. Miscellaneous		Editorial	Editorial

Sources: P/O = Patient/Observed
Questionnaire S/O = Self/Observed

	Minet et al. (1987)	Thomasma (1986)	Kutner (1985)	Evans et al. (1985)	Evans and Manninen (1985)
A. Subject/Controls					
N	81		150	859	
Age	Less than 75 yrs.	Elderly			
Disease	Inoperable non-small cell CA lung		End stage renal disease	End stage renal disease	End stage renal disease
Controls	x		x		
B. Content					
Physical:					
overall	x		x	x	
mobility	x		x		
ADL self-care	x	x			
domestic	x	x			
financial				x	
occupational	x			x	
Psychological:					
overall			x	x	
depression					
anxiety					
anger					
Social Interactions:					
overall					
recreation				x	
effect on the other					
sexual activity					
interest					

Somatic
overall
nausea
pain
GI
sleep
dyspnoea

Angina
x

resp. disease

C. *Procedures*
Source P/O   P   P+O
Questionnaire S/O   O   O
Named QL   Karnofsky   Karnofsky
Validity   x
Reliability   x

D. *Miscellaneous*
RTX alone
combined RTX & chemo   Letter (re 9)   Letter

Sources: P/O = Patient/Observed
Questionnaire S/O = Self/Observed

	Rozenbaum et al. (1985)	Priestman and Baum (1976)	Arora et al. (1986)	Pezim and Nicholls (1985)	Pearlman and Jonson (1985)
A. Subject/Controls					
N	254		55	205 internists	
Age			Elderly		
Disease	Haemodialysis patients	Patient having tx for advanced Br.CA	coronary heart disease	Restorative procto-colectomy with pelvic ileal reservoir	GPs QL & medical decision making
Controls					
B. Content					
Physical:					
overall	x	x	x	x	
mobility		x			
ADL self-care	x	x		x	x
domestic		x			x
financial					
occupational	x				
Psychological:					
overall	x	x		x	
depression					
anxiety		x			
anger					
Social Interaction:					
overall	x			x	
recreation	x	x		x	
effect on other				x	
sexual activity	x			x	
interest	x				

Somatic:				
overall				
nausea		x	x	
pain		x		
GI		x	diet	
sleep	x			
dyspnoea				COPD
C. Procedures				
Source P/O	P	P	P	
Questionnaire S/O	O	P	P	
Named QL	Karnofsky	L.A.S.A.		
Validity	x			
Reliability		x		
D. Miscellaneous			Epidemiological study	One patient assessed by 205 doctors

Sources: P/O = Patient/Observed
Questionnaire S/O = Self/Observed

	Wortman and Yeaton (1985)	Edlund and Tancredi (1985)	Guyatt et al. (1986)	Hunt et al. (1980)	Brown (1987)
A. Subject/Controls					
N	14 trials			162	
Age				Elderly	
Disease	Coronary artery bypass	Many meanings Q/L	Developing a measure for Q/L	4 groups different heart status	Social factors and disease
Controls					
B. Content					
Physical:					
overall				x	x
mobility				x	
ADL self-care					
domestic					
financial					
occupational					
Psychological:					
overall				x	x
depression					
anxiety					
anger					
Social Interaction:					
overall					x
recreation				x	
effect on other					
sexual activity				x	
interest					

	An ideological critique	Q/L in controlled trials	Epicemiological	Sociological
Somatic:				
overall			x	
nausea				
pain Angina			x	
GI				
sleep			x	
dyspnoea				
C. Procedures				
Source P/O			P	
Questionnaire S/O			O	
Named QL Nottingham Heart Profile			x	
Validity		x		
Reliability		x		
D. Miscellaneous				

Sources: P/O = Patient/Observed
Questionnaire S/O = Self Observed

	Harnson (1986)	De Haes and Van Knippenberg (1986)	Croog et al. (1986)	Chessells (1985)	Selby (1985)
A. Subject/Controls					
N			626		
Age	Neonates				
Disease		Review QL cancer pts	Hypertension x	Quality of Life in cancer patients	Measurement QL after cancer Tx
Controls					
B. Content					Examples of measurements and what they measure
Physical:					
overall			x		
mobility					
ADL self-care					
domestic					
financial					
occupational					
Psychological:					
overall			x		
depression					
anxiety					
anger					
Social Interaction:					
overall					
recreation			x		
effect on other					
sexual activity			x		
interest					

Somatic:
  overall
  nausea
  pain
  GI
  sleep
  dyspnoea   x

C. *Procedures*
  Source P/O   P
  Questionnaire S/O   O
  Named QL   Karnofsky
  Validity
  Reliability

D. *Miscellaneous*

Sources: P/O = Patient/Observed
Questionnaire S/O = Self/Observed

	Sugimachi *et al.*	De Haes and Welvaart (1985)	Cribb (1985)	Beu (1985)	Morton *et al.* (1984)
A. Subject/Controls					
N	64	41 (39–63)		25	48
Age					
Disease	CA oesophogus resection & reconstruction	Post surgery for CA Br clinical trial	Response to Calman	Breast cancer patients	Elderly men
Controls					
B. Content					
Physical:					
overall	x	x		x	x
mobility				x	
ADL self-care				x	x
domestic					x
financial					
occupational	x			x	
Psychological:					
overall				x	
depression		x			x
					x
anxiety		Body image		x	DSM.111
anger					
Social Interaction:					
overall					
recreation		x		x	x
effect on other				x	
sexual activity				x	
interest		x			

Somatic:			
overall	x	x Fatigue	x
nausea		x	x
pain		x	x & Discomfort
GI	Appetite, food tolerance dysphagia	x	x
sleep		x	x
dyspnoea		x	x
			Body & life satisfaction
C. Procedures			
Source P/O	P	P	P P
Questionnaire S/O	O	O	P O
Named QL	CPSC	Selby LASA	8 measures
Validity	x	x	x
Reliability	x	x	x
D. Miscellaneous	Tumorectomy & RTX vs radical mastectomy	Compare low or high dose chemo CA Br & Mets	Psychological study

Sources: P/O = Patient/Observed
Questionnaire S/O = Self/Observed

	Kottke (1982)	Flanagan (1982)	Wiklund et al. (1986)	Calman (1984)	Milstein (1985)
A. Subject/Controls					
N					
Age		(30, 50, 70) yr.			
Disease	Disabled				
Controls					
				Calman's Hypothesis Gap E–A	Karnofsky's performance on Prognosis
			QL in clinical trials		
B. Content					
Physical:					
overall	x	x		x	
mobility	x	x		x	
ADL self-care	x	x		x	
domestic	x	x		x	
financial				x	
occupational				x	
Psychological:					
overall	x			x	
depression	x			x	
anxiety	x				
anger	x				
Social Interaction:					
overall	x	x			
recreation	x	x		x	
effect on other	x	x			
sexual activity					
interest					

	Measuring needs 3 Age groups	Editorial	Diet	Bloom's Q/L Scale
Somatic:				
overall			x	
nausea				
pain				
GI				
sleep				
dyspnoea				
C. Procedures				
Source P/O				
Questionnaire S/O				
Named QL				
Validity	x			
Reliability	x			
D. Miscellaneous				

Sources: P/O = Patient/Observed
Questionnaire S/O = Self/Observed

	Bergner *et al.* (1976)	Krupinski (1980)
A. Subject/Controls		
N	278	
Age		
Disease	Sickness impact profile	Australian survey Health QL
Controls		
B. Content		
Physical:		
overall	x	
mobility	x	
ADL self-care	x	
domestic	x	
financial		x
occupational		x
Psychological:		
overall	Emotional feelings	x
depression		
anxiety		
anger		
Social Interaction:		
overall	x	x
recreation	x	x
effect on other	x	
sexual activity	x	
interest		

Somatic:
overall
nausea
pain
GI
sleep
dyspnoea

Nutrition

GI — x (Nutrition)

C. *Procedures*

	Nutrition	
Source P/O	P P	
Questionnaire S/O	P O	
Named QL		
Validity	x	x
Reliability		x

D. *Miscellaneous*

Sources: P/O = Patient/Observed
Questionnaire S/O = Self/Observed

Measuring Health: A Practical Approach
Edited by G. Teeling Smith
© 1988 John Wiley & Sons Ltd

8

Assessment of Treatment in Rheumatoid Arthritis

Morton Paterson
Smith Kline and French Laboratories, Philadelphia

Rheumatoid Arthritis Therapy

Rheumatoid arthritis is an autoimmune disease characterized by inflammation and deterioration of the joints. It typically begins around middle age and attacks women more often than men. The more common symptoms include joint swelling and pain, fatigue, stiffness, and generalized malaise. The disease is not curable but is lifelong and typically progressive with periods of remission and exacerbation. Severe crippling can occur in advanced stages. The prevalence in the United States has been estimated at from 1 to 2 per cent of the population, depending on the diagnostic criteria.

Drug therapy for the initial stages of rheumatoid arthritis has typically involved milder pain killers and non-steroidal anti-inflammatory drugs (NSAIDs), which act directly to reduce inflammation and pain. They are relatively safe oral agents, their most common adverse effect being irritation, sometimes ulceration, of the stomach lining. Their anti-inflammatory efficacy has been demonstrated, but it is unpredictable and often transitory, so that patients frequently try a number of NSAIDs throughout the course of their disease. Therapy for advanced stages of rheumatoid arthritis includes relatively few agents, all more toxic than NSAIDs. A number of these have been considered to be disease-modifying agents (DMARDs) active against the disease process, though they are not curative and therapy is continuous. Some of these agents have quite slow onset of action, perhaps two to four months before effects are seen. Among the slow-acting DMARDs, injectable gold has been proven efficacious in a series of controlled trials and in recent years has become recommended by many as the agent of choice after NSAID therapy has proven inadequate. While NSAIDs are active against inflammation in all types of arthritis, including the far more common osteoarthritis, gold is active only in rheumatoid arthritis. Because of this, the reputation for toxicity of heavy metals, and the skills required to differentially diagnose rheumatoid arthritis, use of gold has been considerably greater among rheumatologists than among non-specialists.

Introduced in the United States in June 1985, auranofin ('Ridaura', SK&F) is the only oral form of gold, containing 0.87 milligrams of the metal in each 3 milligram capsule. Auranofin is indicated only in rheumatoid arthritis and like injectable gold has on average a two to four month delay in onset of efficacy. Recommended initial dosage is two tablets a day. With slow onset of action and no direct effect on joint pain, auranofin needs to be added, at least initially, to existing NSAID therapy. Clinical trials of auranofin (plus background NSAIDs)versus placebo (plus background NSAIDs) done for regulatory approval have demonstrated the incremental efficacy of auranofin at six months and acceptable safety. Although diarrhoea was common among auranofin patients, a considerably greater share of injectable gold patients abandoned therapy because of adverse effects. The prescribing information for auranofin, like the regimen for injectable gold therapy, stipulates regular tests for possible toxicity. Auranofin, then, offers an advance in therapy for rheumatoid arthritis: efficacy comparable to that of the prior standard, with fewer side-effects, and without the inconvenience and pain of intramuscular administration.

The Need for Quality-of-Life Evaluation of Auranofin

During the period of pre-marketing review by the Food and Drug Administration of the auranofin new drug application, Smith Kline & French Laboratories (SK&F) decided to undertake a major additional study of auranofin aimed at defining more completely its effects on patients. There were several reasons. First, the measures of efficacy used in prior trials were the traditional ones: number of swollen joints, number of tender joints, grip strength, time to walk 50 feet, and duration of morning stiffness. While these measures can be applied easily by physicians and together may indicate the severity of the disease process—there is no single measure of severity in rheumatoid arthritis—they do not capture the effects of the pathological process on the health of the patient. While that may sound anomalous, health involves aspects of well-being important to the patient; and these obviously include more than disease-specific pathophysiological observations convenient for diagnosis or medical monitoring—such measures as endoscopically proven lesions in peptic ulcer, wedge pressure in congestive heart failure, spirometric readings in chronic obstructive lung disease, etc. Moreover, in rheumatoid arthritis the incompleteness of traditional measures as indicators even to physicians of 'how well the patient is doing' has been acknowledged by rheumatologists (Bombardier and Tugwell, 1983; Fries, 1985). Thus, while an assessment of the effect of auranofin on the rheumatoid disease process requires traditional observations, an assessment of auranofin's effects on the health of the patient must involve broader observations. These have been called measures of outcome, health status, disability, well being, total health, etc., and more recently have been referred to as quality-of-life measures. That there is no one accepted definition of quality of life does not negate the value of such measures in obtaining a more complete and relevant assessment of drug effects than provided by process measures.

The second reason for undertaking a broader assessment of auranofin was that traditional assessment separates beneficial effects (efficacy), however broadly defined, from adverse effects. Efficacy is presented 'on one side of the ledger', as it were, and safety on the other. The net effect of a drug on the quality of life of the patient experiencing both efficacious effects and perceived adverse effects is not captured in a single metric. Thus, there is no quantified way to determine if the patient is on the whole better off than on alternative therapy. It becomes a matter of judgement by the assessor or physician. With diarrhoea a fairly common experience among auranofin patients, an improved assessment of its effects should incorporate this negative experience and produce, if possible, a net numeric value. Since there were available quality of life measures incorporating adverse as well as therapeutic effects and producing a final number reflecting their net effect, it was decided to use one or more of these measures.

The final reason was that the need to control the costs of medical care is leading increasingly to the application of a cost-effectiveness criterion in the selection and reimbursement of drugs. In the United States, various private health maintenance organizations (HMOs), hospitals, and Medicaid programmes (state plans for the poor and disabled) now forbid use or reimbursement of certain drugs for reasons of cost. When the patient pays out of pocket for drugs, a common practice in the United States, the same concern for value for money is present. While many drugs may 'pay for themselves' by reducing other costs of health care, such as hospitalization or surgery, it is very difficult to prove that new drugs in some classes do this. New analgesics, antihistamines, and antihypertensives, among others, may be of this type, at least in the measurable short term. They may improve patients' well-being but not in ways that reduce discernibly the cost of disease. That is, particularly if they are more expensive than earlier agents or represent add-on therapy, they may in fact increase both drug costs and the total cost of the disease. This is considered a likely effect of much advanced technology and should not be a cause of alarm. It simply means that the benefits to health from the new drug come at a certain increase in net cost. The question then becomes one of cost effectiveness: Does the improvement in health justify the added cost? Is there good value for money? In an era of cost containment this had to be a relevant question in a full assessment of auranofin.

Implications of the Cost-Effectiveness Evaluation

Posing the cost-effectiveness question underlines the incompleteness of traditional, pathophysiological measures of disease and the need for a comprehensive, quality-of-life measure of health. It would be clearly insufficient, for example, for cost-effectiveness evaluation to tell us that auranofin reduced the number of swollen joints in the average patient from 25 to 18 at an added cost of, say (hypothetically), $300. The absence of swollen joints may be relatively unimportant to the patient. It would be more useful to learn that for such a sum the patient improved on broader patient-orientated measures of health, that is, in quality of life. As noted, it is also possible in the case of auranofin that negative experiences of nausea and vomiting might offset whatever gain in quality of life is achieved by the reduction in swollen joints. Thus, while for cost-effectiveness purposes almost any reliable measure in the direction of total health seems preferable to limited pathophysiological measures of disease, the ideal would be a quality-of-life measure including adverse effects. Society, or the patient, is paying for net value. Thus, in opting for a cost-effectiveness evaluation of auranofin, SK&F again faced the need to implement a net measure of quality of life. An attempt was made to express succinctly the type of effectiveness-to-cost relationship that would be produced. The following per-patient ratio was used:

$$\frac{\text{Units of net quality of life gained or lost}}{\text{Cost-of-disease dollars added or saved}}$$

This was recognized as an ideal. It did not strictly rule out the appropriateness of quality-of-life measures that do not include adverse effects. Even these could potentially go beyond traditional measures in quantifying benefits to the patient of auranofin therapy and thereby improve an assessment of its value, even if not reduced to a comprehensive numeric unit.

Selection and Implementation of Quality-of-Life Measures

In medicine these are sometimes called 'instruments' rather than questionnaires because their purpose, like laboratory determinations, is precise measurement and because tasks other than simply answering questions may be involved. When the evaluation was planned, there were not enough published results of the use of quality-of-life instruments to determine whether any would be sensitive to effects of auranofin in a clinical trial (the evaluation method chosen). It was decided that a variety should be used, representing both different types of question-response framework and different dimensions of arthritis and health. Among them would be at least one general health instrument intended to include negative effects of therapy, even though general health instruments were judged likely to be less sensitive to treatment effects than arthritis specific instruments would be. The Quality of Well-Being Questionnaire (Kaplan *et al.*, 1976, 1978; Anderson and Moser 1985) was included partly because its final score expresses a health state in relation to perfect health; and this allows the calculation of years of health (quality-adjusted life years or QALYs) added by treatment. The instruments selected or created for the study are presented in Table 1. Some are arthritis specific, others general health; some assess function, others assess other dimensions of health or arthritis, such as pain; one of the function measures is based on capacity ('can you'), one on performance ('did you'), and another on observation ('try to'). Several of the general health instruments are open to the detection of negative effects. Finally, some of the instruments are preference based. That is, when scored their component questions or items are given different numeric weights reflecting the importance of the item, or preference for positive performance on the item, among patients or other groups as determined by prior preference-weighting studies. Selection of the instruments was based upon the judgement of a consulting group consisting of rheumatologists, a biostatistician, physicians and non-physicians expert in outcome assessment, and a health economist. The goal was comprehensiveness, as no strictly objective method of instrument selection was known.

The number of instruments and the complexity of some had a definite effect on the logistics of evaluation. Most required administration by interviewers. The goal was the collection of quality-of-life data in as accurate and standardized a manner as the collection of laboratory data. This required teaching the mechanics of the instruments and the techniques of interviewing—neutrality, repetition of questions, persistence, etc. Objective interviewing requires a non-involved person, or at least stance, and is not appropriate for busy physicians. Consequently, local interviewers and back-up interviewers, intentionally without medical backgrounds, were hired at each city in which evaluation took place. Identified and hired by SK & F, they reported to and were trained and supervised by Rhode Island Health Services Research (SEARCH). They received forty hours of home study material and four days of centralized training. During the study they tape-recorded their interviews with patients for immediate critique and telephone feedback by SEARCH. SEARCH also processed, quality-controlled and computerized the written response data, which were mailed in weekly. The result was data of excellent quality. Tests by SEARCH of interobserver variability found that the interviewers recorded the same patient's responses with over 97 per cent agreement. Final analysis of study results found that the interviewer-obtained quality of life data showed less variability than did that from the traditional clinical measures administered by the physicians.

The quality of life component of the trial generated various complexities. As usual in clinical trials, the traditional measures by the physician were recorded directly on case report forms, which were collected at intervals by company personnel. Since one of the quality of life instruments (the Quality of Well-Being Questionnaire) asks about patients' symptoms and problems, it was necessary

Table 1. Outcome measures and their major characteristics

Dimension	Administered by interviewer/physician	Minutes to administer	Incorporates adverse effects	Preference-based	Retrospective	Developed/adapted for this trial
Clinical						
Number of joints	yes	2				
Number of swollen joints	yes	2				
50-foot walk time	yes	1				
Duration of morning stiffness	yes	.5				
Grip strength	yes	1				
Pain						
McGill Pain Questionnaire	yes	4				
Pain Ladder Scale	yes	.5				yes
10-Centimetre Pain Line	yes	.5				
Function						
Keitel Assessment	yes	30				
Toronto Activities of Daily Living	yes	15				
Health Assessment Questionnaire	yes	5			yes	
Quality of Well Being Questionnaire	yes	20	yes	yes		
Global Impression						
Arthritis specific:						
Categorical Scale	yes	.5				yes
Ladder Scale	yes	1				yes
Overall Health:						
Ladder Scale, current	yes	.5	yes?			yes
Ladder Scale, six-day mean	yes	1	yes?			yes
10-Centimetre Line, by patient	yes	.5	yes?			yes
10-Centimetre Line, by physician	yes	.5	yes?			yes
Rand Current Health Assessment	yes	3	yes?			yes
Utility						
Patient Utility Measurement Set	yes	30	yes	yes	yes	yes
Standard Gamble Questionnaire	yes	3	yes?	yes		yes
Willingness-to-Pay Questionnaire	yes	3	yes?	yes		yes
Other						
NIMH Depression Questionnaire	yes	5				
Rand General Health Perceptions	yes	7				

for the physician and SK&F to receive duplicates of the interviewer response sheets for this instrument in order to be sure that all adverse experiences were collected by the company. The length of the interview, usually involving several instruments, also required that the participating rheumatologist investigators adjust their scheduling to allow each patient an additional hour of interview time beyond the medical visit time. The interviewer-obtained data were transferred to computer tape by SEARCH; the traditional physician data, after immediate review for adverse effects, were computerized at SK&F. Using Focus, the two tapes were merged at SK&F, then sent to the Harvard School of Public Health for statistical analysis.

Controlled Clinical Trial

The method of evaluation selected was a randomized, placebo-controlled, double-bind clinical trial. This design has become well recognized as the most useful and defensible in establishing the efficacy of drugs. In short, without a control, improvement seen in auranofin patients might be attributed to other causes than the drug itself—suggestion by the physicians, participation in a study, natural remission of the disease, and the like. Placebo, not injectable gold, was chosen as the control because the essential question was not whether auranofin would compare favourably in quality of life or cost with an equally effective but less safe gold regimen, one requiring weekly injections, but whether adding auranofin to a background therapy of NSAIDs would compare favourably with not adding it. Relatively few rheumatoid arthritis patients receive injectable gold. Far more, particularly in earlier stages of the disease and in the larger population of rheumatoid arthritis patients not in the care of rheumatologists, are treated with NSAIDs alone. No safe alternative course is available. The effect of auranofin in this population, where a major decision is whether to initiate gold therapy or not, was clearly more important than discrimination between two forms of gold. Thus, the clinical trial randomized half the patients to auranofin plus continuation of prior NSAIDs and half to placebo plus continuation of prior NSAIDs. The auranofin and placebo capsules were identical, and neither patient nor physician knew who received which until the blind was broken at the end of the trial.

The treatment effect of auranofin was defined as the mean change, on the various measures, of the auranofin patients between the start and end of the trial minus the mean change of the placebo patients. The 'placebo effect' of auranofin is thus subtracted out. As with many drug trials designed to isolate cause and effect, artificialities of the protocol may limit prediction of the effect of the compound under 'normal conditions of use'. (The word 'effectiveness' has been designated for this. 'Efficacy' has been defined as results under 'ideal conditions of use'.) In so far as there is little use of placebo in normal practice, its use in the auranofin evaluation is one such artificiality. In normal practice, the relevant comparison would more likely be between adding known auranofin, perhaps along with the physician's positive suggestion as to its value, versus doing nothing, that is, simply continuing NSAIDs. The placebo group may well do better on measures of outcome than would the do-nothing group, since the latter would be deprived of the suggestive effect of placebo therapy, which can be quite strong. Thus, it was recognized that the treatment effect shown in the trial would satisfy the scientific criteria for cause and effect but might underestimate the degree of effect under normal conditions of use. This was important for the cost-effectiveness evaluation, because that relationship specifically involves effectiveness, not efficacy. Health economists have not sought to define cost-efficacy ratios, since efficacy, if the ideal conditions of use under which it is measured differ from normal conditions of use, is not very meaningful in economic analysis. If the community's resources are to be allocated according to value for money, value must be determined under community conditions of use, not those produced in an experimentally constrained clinical trial. Thus, to the extent that the efficacy of auranofin as determined in the trial would understate the drug's effectiveness, its cost-effectiveness ratio would be less favourable. This was seen as a risk for the trial. However, because the 'real world' alternative, no placebo in the control group, would unblind the trial and leave open to question the very presence of any inherent quality-of-life effect from the compound, the risk was accepted.

Similarly, the costs used in a cost-effectiveness ratio should be those generated under normal conditions of use, not those imposed by the requirements of a carefully monitored trial. All kinds of diagnostic tests and expensive measures of physiological change may be done in a clinical trial—endoscopy in gastritis, for example, to see if stomach lesions are present or have healed—but typically not done in real practice. These not only impose artificial costs but create knowledge on the part of the physician that could lead to atypical therapeutic manoeuvres, which themselves may add or avoid other costs and could alter the very therapeutic outcome under economic investigation, that is, effectiveness. Fortunately, the auranofin protocol required little that differed from normal treatment of rheumatoid arthritis. X-rays and other tests not typical of normal practice were done before the start of the study, and monthly laboratory tests not normally done in NSAID-only patients were required of the placebo as well as the auranofin group. Neither of these artificialities were likely to alter the treatment protocol, and their costs could be eliminated in the cost-effectiveness analysis. The relevant costs to be observed during the trial would be those generated over and above the easily identifiable costs imposed by the protocol. Thus, since comparative costs close to those of normal use and non-use of auranofin could be obtained, meaningful cost-of-disease data were collectable.

While the trial was originally planned to include twelve months of treatment on auranofin or placebo, with a concerted attempt to keep patients on assigned medication for the full term, it became clear that it would be impossible if not unethical to keep non-responding or adversely affected patients on blinded therapy for that length of time. Yet shortening the trial might not allow auranofin, already slow-acting, enough time to exert its full effect. This seemed particularly true in the case of certain cost effects, such as work loss or the use of hired help, which take time to manifest themselves. It was decided that the blinded design could be sustained for six months and that any quality of life effects, if not cost effects, would probably be seen in that period of time. As will be explained below, this was to affect one aspect of the cost-effectiveness evaluation, the QALY calculation, in a way that was not realized when the trial was shortened.

Because the variability of the quality-of-life measures in previous trials was not available, the number of patients required to assure statistical significance, assuming various treatment effects, could not be calculated. It was suggested that a total of 450 patients (225 on auranofin, 225 on placebo) might be necessary for one of the general health instruments; whereas a total of 150 had sufficed for significance on some of the traditional clinical measures used in prior trials of auranofin. It was decided, at some risk to the trial, that 300 patients would be sufficient. To obtain this many required a multicentre trial, and fourteen centres were recruited, twelve in the United States and two in Canada.

Patients were seen two weeks prior to randomization (-2 weeks), at drug start day (0 day) and then at monthly intervals through month 6. The instruments, not all of which could be administered at each visit, were scheduled as shown in Table 2. (If administered at -2 weeks and 0 day, the mean of the two values was used as the baseline).

Number of Patients Analysed

When the trial design was under discussion, it was decided that as much care as possible would be taken to keep patients on assigned medication for six months. If it were necessary to withdraw a patient or break his or her medication code, that patient would continue to be monitored through month 6. The following paragraph to this effect was placed in the study protocol:

> For whatever reason patients exit the double-blind phase of the study prior to six months, they will have the Quality of Life assessment at the originally scheduled intervals, through six months ... and clinical/laboratory evaluations as specified [through month six] in this protocol.

This was unusual in a drug trial. Typically, efficacy data on withdrawn patients are not collected past the point of withdrawal. In this trial, in which comparison of group means was to be based on all or nearly all patients randomized, even if they did not remain on coded medication, it was important to have six months data on as many patients as possible. An alternative approach, basing

Table 2. Frequency of administration of outcome measures

		Study month					
	Baseline	One	Two	Three	Four	Five	Six
Clinical							
Number of tender joints ⎫							
Number of swollen joints ⎪							
50-foot walk time ⎬	x	x	x	x	x	x	x
Duration of morning stiffness ⎪							
Grip strength ⎭							
Pain							
McGill Pain Questionnaire	x	x			x		x
Pain Ladder Scale	x		x		x		x
10-Centimetre Pain Line	x		x		x		x
Function							
Keitel Assessment	x	x					x
Toronto Activities of Daily Living							x
Health Assessment Questionnaire	x	x			x		x
Quality of Well Being Questionnaire	x	x	x		x		x
Global Impression							
Arthritis specific:							
Categorical Scale	x		x		x		x
Ladder Scale	x		x		x		x
Overall Health:							
Ladder Scale, current	x		x		x		x
Ladder Scale, six-day mean	x		x		x		x
10-Centimetre Line, by patient	x		x		x		x
10-Centimetre Line, by physician	x		x		x		x
Rand Current Health Assessment	x				x		
Utility							
Patient Utility Measurement Set						x	
Standard Gamble Questionnaire						x	
Willingness-to-Pay Questionnaire						x	
Other							
NIMH Depression Questionnaire	x	x			x		x
Rand General Health Perceptions	x				x		

Source: Adapted from Bombardier *et al.* (1986).

the efficacy analysis on only those patients completing the study on assigned blinded medication, though common in drug studies, was considered to be unacceptable. While there are arguments for the latter method when attempting to define the presence of inherent activity in a compound, it seemed particularly suspect in cost-effectiveness analysis. This is because while withdrawn patients may perhaps be ignored in an efficacy analysis, ignoring their costs after early withdrawal would add considerable uncertainty to the cost side of the effectiveness-cost ratio. (This issue of a definition of cost-effectiveness in the context of a controlled clinical trial is one that health economists might usefully address.)

In any case, through the attention of the study planners and the cooperation of the participating centres, the completion problem was largely obviated. As noted by Bombardier, Ware and co-workers in the first detailed report of study results (Bombardier *et al.*, 1986), of 311 eligible patients randomized only 8 were withdrawn from the study drug and lost to follow up before three months; and of the remaining 303 patients, 294 were followed into the sixth month. The efficacy analysis was based on the 303 patients completing at least three months of therapy, since auranofin has an onset of effect about three months after initiation. The values for the nine patients lost to follow-up between months 3 and 6 were their last values recorded.

Adverse Effects

Analysis of safety was based on 309 of the 311 eligible patients randomized, two having been lost to follow-up immediately after randomization. As expected from prior auranofin studies, diarrhoea occurred significantly more often in the auranofin group (59 per cent of that group) than in the placebo group (19 per cent), as shown in Table 3. While in 24 per cent of auranofin-treated patients the diarrhoea was moderate to severe, requiring at least temporary discontinuance, in only 4 per cent did it require permanent discontinuance of the drug. Diarrhoea tended to present early in the course of treatment—30 per cent of those auranofin patients with diarrhoea being affected in the first month—so that by month 6 the cumulative proportion of patients with at least one episode was levelling. In addition, significantly more patients in the auranofin group (21 per cent of that group) experienced abdominal pain than did placebo patients (11 per cent). Certain laboratory anomalies were more common in the auranofin group.

Beneficial Effects

As noted, for most measures the treatment effect (efficacy or effectiveness) was defined as the difference between the average change of the auranofin group between baseline and month 6 and the average change of the placebo group. (On

Table 3. Adverse events by treatment groups ($n = 309$)

	Placebo ($n = 152$)		Auranofin ($n = 157$)		
	Number	%	Number	%	P value
Diarrhoea	29	19	93	59	<0.0001
Rash	31	20	37	24	0.50
Digestive[a]	37	24	48	31	0.22
Abdominal pain	16	11	33	21	0.01
Oral ulcers/stomatitis	18	12	17	11	0.78
Pruritus	10	7	20	13	0.07
Headache, general	10	7	19	12	0.10
Proteinuria[b]	1	0.7	5	3.2	0.22
Anemia[c]	1	0.7	1	0.6	1.00
Leukopenia[d]	3	2.0	1	0.6	0.37
Thrombocytopenia[e]	1	0.7	2	1.3	1.00
Serum glutamic oxaloacetic transaminase increase[f]	1	0.7	6	0.8	0.12
Alkaline phosphatase increase[f]	0	0.0	4	2.6	0.12
Blood urea nitrogen increase[g]	2	1.3	6	3.8	0.28

[a] Includes nausea, vomiting, gastrointestinal disorder (general).

[b] 2+ or higher by dipstick, or 1 g per 24 hours.

[c] Hemoglobin more than 10 per cent below investigator's lower limit of normal, or at least 3 g/dl drop from baseline.

[d] Less than $3,000/mm^3$.

[e] Less than $100,000/mm^3$.

[f] More than twice investigator's upper limit of normal.

[g] At least 20 per cent above investigator's upper limit of normal. or at least 30 mg/dl.

Source: Reproduced from Bombardier *et al.* (1986).

four measures, Toronto Activities of Daily Living, Patient Utility Measurement Set, Standard Gamble, and Willingness to Pay, no baseline observation was made and the treatment effect was ascertained at month 5 or 6 of treatment.) In sum, this difference was positive for auranofin on virtually all measures. As seen in Table 4, on most measures the treatment effect attained reasonably high levels of statistical significance. Some were highly significant.

Traditional Clinical Measures

Overall results on the traditional measures, showing a consistent trend toward greater improvement in the auranofin group, were similar to those of prior auranofin trials. The auranofin patients at six months reduced on average the number of their tender joints by about three more joints (-7.3 vs -4.5 joints) and their swollen joints by about two more joints (-5.5 vs -3.6 joints) than did the placebo-treated patients. Also, the auranofin patients reduced their time to walk 50 feet by about one and a third more seconds than did the placebo patients, who actually increased their walk time (-0.74 vs $+0.61$ seconds); and they reduced their experience of morning stiffness by sixteen more minutes than did the placebo group (-28 vs -12 minutes). Finally, at six months, the average auranofin patient could squeeze up more millimetres of mercury in the grip strength test than he or she could at baseline, whereas the average placebo patient could squeeze up fewer millimetres than at baseline ($+13$ vs -2 millimetres). The lower levels of statistical significance for walking time and duration of morning stiffness reflected a high measurement error for these variables from visit to visit (Bombardier *et al.*, 1986). Normally, these five clinical measures, traditionally used in attempts to represent the severity of a disease process not defined by any single objective measure, would supply the main, if not sole, quantification of the positive effect of auranofin therapy. Against this an estimate of the degree of negative experience from diarrhoea or abdominal pain would be weighed judgmentally by the physician —perhaps by the interested patient as well, and possibly, in today's environment, by the health plan manager. Clearly, in a trade-off decision to treat with auranofin, a central question was whether improvements observed by the traditional measures extended to improvements in performance and other outcomes valued in daily life.

Measures of Pain

Effect on pain further defines the overall effect of auranofin. The drug has no direct effect on the pain of inflammation, as have NSAIDS, so that evidence of pain reduction was not assumed when the trial was planned. An indirect effect on pain did occur, however, as is apparent in the scores of three pain measures used. Perhaps because of a less than direct effect, the degree of statistical significance seen with the pain measures is not as high overall as that of the traditional measures. On the McGill Pain Questionnaire (Melzak, 1975), auranofin patients selected fewer higher-scoring (more 'severe') words to describe their present pain, resulting in a score improvement 2.4 points better than that of the placebo patients (-8 vs -5.6). This questionnaire has a score range from 78 (worst) to 0. Though the score changes at six months were positive (towards zero) and auranofin performed better than placebo by 2.4 points ($P = 0.02$), without experience with other applications of the measure, it is difficult to tell how important to patients is a reduction of 8 and 5.6 on this scale, or how important is a difference of 2.4. The Pain Ladder Scale, constructed for this trial and calibrated in equal degrees from 'most severe imaginable pain' (0) to 'no pain' (10), is perhaps more straightforward. Auranofin patients improved about a third of a step more than did placebo patients ($+0.96$ vs $+0.61$ degrees). Statistical significance, however, was less than with the McGill questionnaire. A more familiar type of instrument was the non-calibrated visual analogue scale or 10-centimetre Pain Line (Scott and Huskisson, 1976; Dickson and Bird, 1981)—from 'excruciating' (10, right end) to 'none' (0, left end). A cross is placed on the line to indicate the degree of joint pain currently experienced. This simple measure proved the most sensitive of the pain measures

Table 4. Results of outcome measures at month 6 ($n = 303$)[a]

	Possible range (worst to best)	Placebo ($n = 149$) Baseline	Change	Auranofin ($n = 154$) Baseline	Change	Treatment effect	P value[b]
Clinical							
Number of tender joints		26	−4.5	25	−7.3	−2.8	.01
Number of swollen joints		22	−3.6	21	−5.5	−1.9	.01
50-foot walk time (seconds)		15	0.61	15	−0.74	−1.35	.11
Duration of morning stiffness (minutes)		133	−12	119	−28	−16	.1
Grip strength (mm Hg)		113	−2	113	13	15	.02
Pain							
McGill Pain Questionnaire	78–0	23	−5.6	22	−8	−2.4	.02
Pain Ladder Scale	0–10	5.5	0.61	5.5	0.96	0.35	.09
10-Centimetre Pain Line	10–0	5.3	−0.91	5.3	1.44	0.53	.01
Function							
Keitel Assessment	98–0	30	1.7	30	−1.5	−3.2	.003
Toronto Activities of Daily Living	−4–1	—	0.00[c]	—	0.02[c]	0.02	.02
Health Assessment Questionnaire	3–0	1.39	−0.17	1.4	−0.31	−0.14	.01
Quality of Well Being Questionnaire	0–1	0.6	−0.001	−0.599	0.023	0.024	.005

Global Impression						
Arthritis Specific:						
Categorical Scale	1–5	2.8	0.31	2.9	0.65	0.34	<.001
Ladder Scale	0–10	5	0.59	4.8	0.98	0.39	.11
Overall Health:						
Ladder Scale, current	0–10	6.1	0.39	6	0.65	0.26	.19
Ladder Scale, six-day mean	0–10	5.8	0.35	5.7	0.87	0.52	.007
10-Centimetre Line, by patient	0–10	5.6	0.51	5.5	0.89	0.38	.1
10-Centimetre Line, by physician	0–10	6.2	0.46	6.2	0.58	0.12	2
Rand Current Health Assessment	9–45	22	0.51	22	1.82	1.31	.01
Utility						
Patient Utility Measurement Set	0–100	—	9.9[c]	—	20.9[c]	11	.002
Standard Gamble Questionnaire	100–0	—	30[d]	—	23[d]	−7	.07
Willingness-to-Pay Questionnaire	100–0	—	23[d]	—	21[d]	−2	.79
Other						
NIMH Depression Questionnaire	60–0	15	−4.1	15	−3.3	0.8	.54
Rand General Health Perceptions	0–110	66	−0.07	67	0.52	0.59	.32

[a] Except Utility measures, where *n* varied from 217 to 243.

[b] Significance level of the treatment effect determined by analysis of covariance adjusting for baseline valued of age, sex, centre, functional class, and the variable tested (except where the variable tested was not observed at baseline).

[c] Derived change score: no value obtained at baseline; recorded retrospectively at month 5 or 6 from patient's comparison of baseline and current states.

[d] Not a change score: no baseline value obtained or calculated.

Adapted from Bombardier *et al.* 1986.

to the treatment effect of auranofin (p = 0.01). Again, one is not sure of the importance of the changes observed.

Measures of Function

The measures of function selected for the trial, while all directed to this well-acknowledged dimension of arthritis, differ from each other fundamentally in their attempt to encompass the overall health of the patient, to capture adverse effects, and to allow for preference or importance—that is, the relative preference of the patient for performance on the different items rated. The Keitel Assessment (Eberl *et al.*, 1976) involves 23 range-of-motion tasks (e.g. touch shoulder with hand) performed by the patient. The interviewer records the difficulty with which each is performed, resulting in a total score from 98 (worst) to 0. Between baseline and month 6, auranofin patients improved their score by an average of -1.5 points, whereas placebo patients worsened by $+1.7$ points. (The difference was highly significant statistically at p = 0.003.) The score obviously represents a physical or bodily subdimension of function and is essentially additive (weighting equally performance on each task), rather than preference based.

The Toronto Activities of Daily Living Questionnaire (Helewa *et al.* 1982) as used in this trial, an arthritis-specific instrument, scores to what extent performance of activities in twenty-one areas of daily living has changed, in the patient's opinion, since the start of therapy. These retrospectively orientated change questions were administered at month 6. Responses can range from ('a lot worse') to ('a lot better'), with an overall score range from -4 (worst) to $+1$. The six-month value for the auranofin group was 0.02, and 0.00 for the placebo group (p = 0.02). While the scoring system is not preference-weighted and is somewhat complex, a higher change score represents concrete improvements in the performance of a wide variety of daily tasks, ranging from basic self- care to social and work-related interactions. As such, the instrument captures a broad aspect of quality of life in considerable detail.

The Health Assessment Questionnaire or HAQ (Fries *et al.*, 1982; Fries, 1985), another arthritis-specific instrument of the activities-of-daily-living type, specifies eight areas of daily function (e.g. hygiene) each with two to three activities (e.g. take a tub bath). The patient reports his or her difficulty in performing each activity during the past week, and the degree of difficulty is scored from 3 ('unable to do') to 0 ('without any difficulty'); the lower values are raised if aids, devices, or help from another are needed. The overall score ranged from 3.00 (worst) to 0. The HAQ was administered at baseline and throughout the trial. Auranofin patients improved by an average of -0.31 on this measure, placebo patients by -0.17 (p = 0.01). The greater average improvement of -0.14 points in the auranofin group is about the same as would be produced by a change from the ability to walk outdoors on level

Table 5. Quality of Well-Being Questionnaire: function levels

Level No.	Level definition	Weight
	Mobility Scale (MOB)	
5	No limitations for health reasons	−0.000
4	Did not drive a car, health-related (younger) than 16 yr); did not ride in a car as usual for age, health-related, and/or did not use public transportation, health-related; or had or would have used more help than usual for age to use public transportation, health-related.	−0.082
2	In hospital, health-related.	−0.090
	Physical Activity Scale (PAC)	
4	No limitations for health reasons.	−0.000
3	In wheelchair, moved or controlled movement of wheelchair without help from someone else; or had trouble or did not try to lift, stoop, bend over, or use stairs or inclines, health-related, and/or limped, used a cane, crutches, or walker, health-related; and/or had any other physical limitation in walking, or did not try to walk as far or as fast as others the same age are able; health-related	−0.060
1	In wheelchair, did not move or control the movement of wheelchair without help from someone else, or in bed, chair, or couch for most or all of the day, health-related.	−0.077
	Social Activity Scale (SAC)	
5	No limitations for health reasons.	−0.000
4	Limited in other (e.g. recreational) role activity, health-related.	−0.061
3	Limited in major (primary) role activity, health-related.	−0.061
2	Performed no major role activity, health-related, but did perform self-care activities.	−0.061
1	Performed no major role activity, health-related, and did not perform or had more help than usual in performance or one or more self-care activities, health-related.	−0.106

Source: Adapted from Anderson and Moser (1985)

group with much difficulty to the ability to walk outdoors on level ground with some difficulty, or from getting out of bed with much difficulty to getting out of bed with some difficulty; either of these changes in degree of function would produce a −0.125 improvement in HAQ score. With this translation to one specific improvement in daily function we have a more concrete representation of treatment effect. Again, the instrument assigns equal preference weights to all activities. As in all the results presented so far, negative experiences from adverse effects are not incorporated.

The Quality of Well-Being Questionnaire or QWB (Kaplan *et al.*, 1976, 1978) is designed to measure functional disability in all diseases. The patient is asked what he or she did or did not do because of health on each of the last six days. The responses classify the patient into a given level of ability within three areas of performance, listed in Table 5 (Anderson and Moser, 1985). A predetermined weight is assigned to each level. The QWB also asks about symptoms and health problems, each with the predetermined weight shown in Table 6 (Anderson and Moser, 1985). The worse the symptom/problem or disability, the higher its weight. All weights recorded for a patient are added and the sum subtracted from 1.000, representing full health (i.e. 0 disability and 0 symptoms), so that the lower the resulting score the worse is the patient's well-being. As seen in Table 6, diarrhoea reported by a patient in the trial would lower that patient's score by 0.290. Ordinarily, when the QWB is scored the values assigned to each level of disability or symptom/problem are those determined from prior studies of preferences in a normal population. In this trial, the rheumatoid arthritis patients themselves were given preference sorting and ranking tasks in order to determined the values to be used. These values agreed closely with those from the prior studies (Balaban *et al.*, 1986). Thus, the QWB not only includes adverse effects of therapy but weights all response items according to preference or importance. The QWB score is thus a more comprehensive measure of effect than any other instrument so far discussed.

Despite qualms when the trial was planned about the possible insensitivity of the QWB to changes in rheumatoid arthritis patients, the instrument proved highly sensitive to treatment effect. At baseline, auranofin and placebo groups averaged virtually the same on the QWB— 0.599 and 0.600 respectively on the scale from 0 to 1.000 (death to full health). By month 6, the auranofin group had improved by 0.023, and the placebo group worsened slightly by -0.001. The difference is highly significant statistically ($p = 0.005$). As was apparent in the discussion of the instruments above, one of the problems with quality-of-life scores is whether a particular change in score is clinically important. This question seems accentuated in the case of the QWB by the small numeric range of the scale. However, as can be seen in Table 5, the 0.024 treatment effect observed in the trial represents, approximately, the equivalent of an improvement by the average auranofin patient from using a wheelchair with help (PAC level 1) to walking with physical limitations (PAC level 3), a $+0.017$ change on the QWB. Improving from being hospitalized (MOB level 2) to using public transportation with help (MOB level 4) would produce a $+0.280$ change on the QWB, again about as much as the $+0.024$ observed in the trial. As noted, the average score improvement of $+0.024$ in the trial is net; that is, it includes adverse drug experiences such as diarrhoea. Again, the effect of auranofin is more apparent from a thorough understanding of the scoring system of the QWB instrument and translation to a single specific improvement in function.

Table 6. Quality of Well-Being Questionnaire: symptoms/problems

S/P No.	Symptom/problem	Weights
1	Death (not on respondent's card).	−0.727
2	Loss of consciousness such as seizure (fits), fainting, or coma (out cold or knocked out).	−0.407
3	Burn over large areas of face, body, arms, or legs.	−0.367
4	Pain, bleeding, itching, or discharge (drainage) from sexual organs—does not include normal menstrual (monthly) bleeding.	−0.349
5	Trouble learning, remembering, or thinking clearly.	−0.340
6	Any combination of one or more hands, feet, arms, or legs either missing, deformed (crooked), paralysed (unable to move), or broken—includes wearing artificial limbs or braces.	−0.333
7	Pain, stiffness, weakness, numbness, or other discomfort in chest, stomach (including hernia or rupture), side, neck, back, hips or any joints of hands, feet, arms, or legs.	−0.299
8	Pain, burning, bleeding, itching, or other difficulty with rectum, bowel movements, or urination (passing water).	−0.292
9	Sick or upset stomach, vomiting or loose bowel movement, with or without fever, chills, or aching all over.	−0.290
10	General tiredness, weakness, or weight loss.	−0.259
11	Cough, wheezing, or shortness of breath with or without fever, chills, or aching all over.	−0.257
12	Spells of feeling upset, being depressed, or of crying.	−0.257
13	Headache, or dizziness, or ringing in ears, or spells of feeling hot, or nervous, or shaky.	−0.244
14	Burning or itching rash on large areas of face, body, arms, or legs.	−0.240
15	Trouble talking, such as lisp, stuttering, hoarseness, or being unable to speak.	−0.237
16	Pain or discomfort in one or both eyes (such as burning or itching) or any trouble seeing after correction.	−0.230
17	Overweight for age and height or skin defect of face, body, arms, or legs, such as scars, pimples, warts, bruises, or changes in colour.	−0.186
18	Pain in ear, tooth, jaw, throat, lips, tongue; several missing or crooked permanent teeth—includes wearing bridges or false teeth; stuffy, runny nose; or any trouble hearing—includes wearing a hearing aid.	−0.170
19	Taking medication or staying on a prescribed diet for health reasons	−0.144
20	Wore eyeglasses or contact lenses.	−0.101
21	Breathing smog or unpleasant air.	−0.101
22	No symptom or problem (not on respondent's card).	−0.000
23	Standard symptom/problem.	−0.257

Source: Adapted from Anderson and Moser (1985)

Global Measures

Global measures ask the patient simply to designate directly an impression of his or her health state. Global arthritis measures focus on that disease only. In the Arthritis Categorical Scale the patient selects one of five possible responses from 'very poor' to 'very good' to describe his or her arthritis 'condition today'. Scores range from 1 (worst) to 5. On this range the auranofin group improved by +0.65 and the placebo group by +0.31. This simple 'how are you today' type measure had the distinction of producing the highest degree of statistical significance of all measures of any type used in the trial ($p = <0.001$). The Arthritis Ladder Scale shows 10 equal degrees of arthritis activity from 'most severe problems' (0, bottom) to 'no problems' (10, top). The patient selects the degree of arthritis 'activity' experienced on each of the past six days, and a six-day average score from 0 to 10 is calculated. The auranofin group showed a mean improvement of +0.98 degrees on this scale, the placebo group +0.59 ($p = 0.11$). Global overall health measures are intended to capture total health. The Overall Health Ladder Scale, Current, shows 10 equal degrees of health from 'least desirable' (0, bottom) to 'most desirable' (10, top). The patient selects the degree indicating his or her current 'health situation'. Scores can range from 0 to 10. On this scale, the auranofin group improved +0.65 degrees, the placebo group +0.39 ($p = 0.19$). The Overall Health Ladder Scale, Six-Day Mean, is similar to the above, but the score is an average of the responses for each of the past six days. The auranofin group improved +0.87 degrees, the placebo group +0.35 ($p = 0.007$). The 10-Centimetre Line Overall Health Scale, by Patient, is another visual-analogue, non-calibrated line labelled 'poor' (0, left end) to 'perfect' (10, right end). The patient makes a cross to indicate his or her 'overall health status'. Auranofin patients averaged an improvement of +0.89 centimetres, the placebo group +0.51 centimetres ($p = 0.1$). The 10-Centimetre Overall Health Scale, by Physician, is identical to the above, except the patient's health status is indicated by the physician. Auranofin patients averaged an improvement of +0.58 centimetres, placebo patients +0.46 ($p = 0.2$). All the above measures were constructed for the trial. The Rand Current Health Assessment (Brook *et al.*, 1979), an already available instrument, lists 19 statements about current health (e.g. 'I'm as healthy as anybody I know' or 'Doctors say that I am now in poor health'), which the patient classifies as 'definitely true', 'definitely false', or 'don't know'. The differently valued responses are combined to give a score from 9 (worst) to 45. Auranofin patients averaged an improvement of +1.82, placebo patients +0.51 ($p = 0.01$). While it may seem repetitive to have used so many similar global measures in the trial, all of which showed a positive effect for auranofin, when the trial was planned it was not known if any of the global measures would be sensitive to treatment effect. It seemed prudent to try various approaches.

Because the global arthritis measures are directed specifically to that disease, adverse effects of therapy such as diarrhoea cannot be considered to be incorporated. However, the global overall health measures are not disease specific and theoretically allow the patient to consider experience with adverse effects. The patient is not directed to consider this, however, so that it is not clear whether the global overall health measures are in fact measures of net effect. Another problem with global measures is their lack of component items, making it impossible to learn anything about what has changed in the condition or life of the patient. No translation to a concrete behavioural situation is possible nor are any of the ranges anchored between full health and some other known state, such as death (as is the QWB), so that there are no fixed points of reference for the scores. Even if there were such 'anchors', it would not be correct to assume the ordinal distances on the scales represented equal degrees of severity. Finally, for related reasons, importance or preference is not captured. In sum, it is virtually impossible to know whether the treatment effect observed on any one of the global measures is important. Because of these problems, global measures, sometimes used in clinical evaluations, are typically taken less seriously than are traditional measures of disease process.

Utility Measures

Since these types of measures are somewhat difficult to explain, it would be well to quote the description of them by Bombardier, Ware *et al.* (1986):

> Utility measures quantify the worth or value to a person of his or her health state by determining the risks or sacrifices he or she would undertake in order to improve it. The assumption is that patients with better health will accept less risk or sacrifice less in order to improve than will more severely affected patients. By varying the risk or sacrifice in quantitative terms, a numeric value for the 'utility' of the health state is derived.

Three instruments of this type, each developed or adapted for the trial, were employed, each in the fifth month. They were administered to from 217 to 243 patients, depending on the instrument—not to all patients, as some had finished the trial before these instruments were ready for use. The most complex of the three was the Patient Utility Measurement Sert (PUMS), designed by Pauker, McNeil, and Torrance (Pauker *et al.*, in preparation).

Again, it would be difficult to improve on Bombardier, Ware *et al.*'s summary of the PUMS (1986): '[It] elicits the patient's perception of his or her current state at the beginning of the trial and relative to a state of full health. Negative experiences, including adverse effects of drug treatment, are mentioned for inclusion in the patient's consideration of the current and pre-trial health states.' The authors' Appendix elaborates:

Three health states as perceived by the patient—current, pre-trial, and full health—are initially related to each other on a traditional visual analogue scale labeled 'health' at the top (100) points. The states are then further related in the context of three assessment techniques—the lottery, the modified time trade-off, and the standard time trade-off. Each involves a hypothetic new treatment that will make the patient fully healthy in return for varied degrees of risk or sacrifice. For simplicity, we assume a male patient whose condition has improved during the trial. (For patients who believe their pre-trial state was better than their current state, the terms of the scenarios are inverted.) In the LOTTERY scenario, the patient chooses between continuing permanently at his current level of health or receiving a hypothetic new treatment that has some percentage chance (p) of returning him permanently to the pre-trial level of health and a corresponding chance $(1 - p)$ of producing permanent full health. A full range of chances is offered to the patient. The better his current health, the lower the chance of returning to his pre-trial level will be acceptable in order to have the chance of full health. In the MODIFIED TIME TRADE-OFF scenario, the choice is again between continuing at the current level of health or receiving a hypothetic treatment; however, the treatment, instead of producing a permanent pre-trial or healthy state, produces these states for different numbers of months each year. In the STANDARD TIME TRADE-OFF scenario, the patient chooses between surviving at his current level of health for the rest of his normal life expectancy (specific to the patient's age) or receiving a hypothetic treatment that will give him full health but shorten his life expectancy—i.e., the patient may trade remaining years of life for full health while living. The more the patient has improved, the fewer remaining years of life at his current level of health will be sacrificed in return for full health while surviving. This scenario is repeated with a choice between receiving the same type of hypothetic treatment or returning to and surviving at the pre-trial level of health for the rest of normal life expectancy. In all scenarios the variables—percent chance, months per year, and years of life— are ascribed to the hypothetic treatment in a converging 'ping pong' manner until the patient feels indifferent, i.e., believes the treatment would be as acceptable as continuing at his current level of health (or, as in the last case, at the pre-trial level). The patient's score is produced at the indifference point. From the results of the visual analogue scale, the modified time trade-off, and the lottery, a change score is calculated for the patient, representing the difference between his pre-trial and current health states. Combining this score with results of the standard time trade-off produces an overall score for the patient's current state of health compared with his recollected baseline state. This score is expressed as a number of points on a scale of 0 to 100.

For the auranofin group this change score was $+20.9$, for the placebo group $+9.9$ ($p = 0.002$). These represent improvements of 37 per cent and 16 per cent, respectively, over the retrospectively determined pre-trial values. Since these are net treatment effects, that is, they incorporate adverse effects, and are by design completely preference- or utility-based, they should represent at least as fully as the QWB does the value of the auranofin effect to the patient. In fact, it can be argued that because the PUMS elicits the preferences of each individual patient as an inherent part of his or her score the PUMS is more meaningfull than the QWB, which uses average preference weights based on a group of patients. A difficulty in understanding the PUMS is created by its extremely complex system of score calculation. Perhaps it is best to focus on the final score as a number of units of quality of life, as defined by the patient, where 100 is perfect health and 0 is none. Thus, the effect of auranofin was a 20.9 point improvement on a 100-point quality-of-life continuum, 11 points greater than the improvement of the placebo group.

The second of the three utility measures in the trial was also administered in month 5.

> The Standard Gamble Questionnaire asks the patient to choose simply between his or her current state and a hypothetic treatment with systematically varied chances of causing either complete cure or death. Change is not measured, as no reference to the pre-trial state is made. The higher the risk accepted by the patient, the worse his or her condition is considered to be. Results are expressed as the maximal percent chance of death (0 to 100) accepted by the patient. (Bombardier *et al.*, 1986)

It was perhaps unrealistic to expect such a present-orientated measure, that is, one which neither observed the pre-trial state nor made reference to it retrospectively, to be sensitive to treatment effect. However, the auranofin patients were willing on average to accept a 23 per cent chance of death to be cured, the placebo patients a 30 per cent chance of death—indicating that placebo patients were in worse condition at the end of the trial. The treatment effect was not highly significant statistically ($p = 0.07$).

Finally, the Willingness to Pay Questionnaire, also administered in month 5, elicits the

> share the patient's household income he or she would pay for a hypothetic cure of arthritis. Discussion and revision of answers are permitted. No reference to the pre-trial condition is made. The greater the share the patient would pay, the worse his or her condition is considered to be. Results are expressed as percent of income (0 to 100 percent) (Bombardier *et al.*, 1986)

Results were essentially the same for the auranofin and placebo groups, 23 per cent of income versus 21 per cent respectively ($p = 0.79$). The value of willingness-to-pay questions is controversial. The nature and performance of this instrument, and of the Standard Gamble Questionnaire, is discussed in detail by Thompson, their developer for use in this trial (Thompson, 1986).

Other Measures

These were not selected as measures of drug *per se* but as items of interest which might change along with the measures above. The National Institute of Mental Health (NIMH) Depression Questionnaire (Radloff, 1977; Husaini *et al.*, 1979) elicits on how many of the last seven days the patient experienced twenty feelings or attitudes indicative of depression. The number is transformed into a score from 60 (worst) to 0. Auranofin patients improved on average -3.3, placebo patients -4.1. This is the only measure among all those used in the trial on which the placebo group improved by a greater amount than did the auranofin group; but the difference is insignificant ($p = 0.54$). The Rand General Health Perceptions Questionnaire (Brook *et al.*, 1979) contains 36 statements that may reflect the patient's feelings and attitudes towards his or her past and future health care and outlook. As such it was not expected to change significantly during the course of the trial. True or false responses are combined to give an overall score from 0 (worst) to 110. The auranofin group improved by $+0.52$; the placebo group worsened by -0.07. Again, the difference was not significant ($p = 0.32$).

Analysis of Composite Scores

With so many measures it seemed possible that auranofin might produce a significant positive treatment effect on some measures and insignificant or negative (less than placebo) treatment effect on other measures. To avoid this problem of multiple comparisons, some of which might be favourable by chance, and generally to simplify summarization of results, it was decided prior to analysis of the auranofin results that the measures should be divided into four logical groups: clinical (traditional), functional, pain, and global. Within each group a composite score was calculated by dividing each component outcome by its observed baseline standard deviation, changing sign if necessary so that a larger score represented improvement, and taking the mean of these standardized outcomes as the composite score. (This meant that measures without baseline observations would not be included in the composites. Thus, the Toronto Activities of Daily Living Questionnaire and the utility measures were not part of the composite measures. The NIMH Depression Questionnaire and the Rand General Health Perceptions Questionnaire were also excluded.) The primary hypotheses of the study were that auranofin would produce improvement in each group. Furthermore, each hypothesis would need to be proven at the 0.0125 level (two-sided) of significance or better, which would equal a level of at least 0.05 for the study as a whole. As seen in Table 7, the treatment effect of auranofin met or exceeded the 0.0125 level on three of the four composite measures—clinical, functional, and global—and trended in the same direction of the pain composite.

Table 7. Results of composite measures at month 6

Composite	Placebo		Auranofin		Treatment effect	P value
	Baseline	Change	Baseline	Change		
Clinical	−1.6	0.16	−1.5	0.35	0.19	0.003
Pain	−0.63	0.48	−0.72	0.74	0.26	0.021
Functional	0.96	0.05	0.98	0.28	0.23	0.001
Global	3.6	0.27	3.5	0.5	0.23	0.007

Source: Adapted from Bombardier *et al.* (1986).

Cost-effectiveness Analysis

A utilization of services questionnaire was administered at baseline and at month 6 of the trial. Constructed for the trial, it asked the patient about office visits, hospitalizations, purchase of aids and devices. physiotherapy, consumption of arthritis-related drugs, work status, use of hired help, and other events which might contribute to cost of disease. In the case of hospitalizations, the patient reports were verified by a check of the hospital records. Local unit costs for each type of event were obtained and applied to the event frequency reported during the trial. The cumulated six-month costs of the auranofin and placebo patients were then compared, and the difference was taken as due to auranofin. As noted above, cost events imposed by the trial protocol were excluded from the analysis. Results of the cost comparison and the cost-effectiveness analysis will be reported by Thompson and cannot be given here (Thompson, forthcoming).

For present purposes, results of the cost comparison will be *hypothesized* only, then used with the actual quality-of-life outcomes above to explore certain issues of method and interpretation that arise from the trial. Our hypothesized result of the cost comparison is that the auranofin group, largely because of the costs of auranofin itself and associated monthly monitoring visits, neither of which would be borne by a placebo-treated group, generates $300 more in costs over the six-month period than does the placebo-treated group. It could well be that the auranofin group had lower costs than the placebo group because of reduced hospitalizations, use of hired help, or other changes due to improved health; but the more useful hypothesis for exploration of cost-effectiveness analysis is that during the relatively short period of the trial auranofin increased net cost as it increased quality of life. This clearly poses the value-for-money question.

The effectiveness value for the numerator of the effectiveness-to-cost ratio could be any of the outcomes measured. Using treatment effect as measured by grip strength (a +13 mm Hg improvement by month 6 for the auranofin group minus a −2 mm Hg deterioration for the placebo group) would give 15 mm Hg/$300 as the effectiveness-cost ratio. More indicative of total health gain at six months would be the result on the Health Assessment Questionnaire (HAQ) functional instrument: −0.14 points on the 3.00 (worst) to 0 scale, giving −0.14 HAQ units/$300. As noted above, this improvement can be concretized within the HAQ framework as the equivalent of the ability to get out of bed with much difficulty minus the ability to get out of bed with some difficulty. The Quality of Well-Being Questionnaire, including adverse effects and offering preference weighted scores, should be particularly useful in assessing treatment effect in a value-for-money analysis. The QWB result at six months was a treatment effect of +0.024 on a range from 0 to 1.000 (full health), giving a ratio of +0.024 QWB units/$300. This represents a gain approximately equivalent to one of improving from being in the hospital to being able to use public transportation with help. Given the death-to-health, 0 to 1.000 range of the QWB, the gain can also be expressed as a percentage of full health, giving the ratio 2.4 per cent full health/$300. The quality-of-life gain on the Patient Utility Measurement Set (PUMS), 11 points on a 0 to 100 range, might be expressed as 11 per cent full health/$300. This average gain might be concretized in terms of a number of years of life the patient would be willing to give up in order to be healthy while living, or in terms used by other scenarios in the PUMS.

QALY Calculations

The QWB was of interest when the trial was planned because it allowed the calculation of the number of QALYs (a year of life in full health) gained from use of auranofin. If a patient experiences a gain of 2.4 per cent of full health for a full year, that patient has gained 2.4 per cent of a QALY. Single patients rarely gain a whole QALY, as that would be the equivalent of living a year in full health instead of living it in a coma or being dead. (However, if 100 patients were to live for a year at a level of health 2.4 per cent better than otherwise, 2.4 QALYs would have been gained by that group, at the total added cost generated by the group.) Costs to add a QALY have been estimated at from $3,000 or less for instituting a screening programme for phenylketonuria (Bush *et al.*, 1973) to over $85,000 for certain uses of leukocyte transfusion (Rosenshein *et al.*, 1980). If $300 produced a gain of 2.4 per cent of full health on the QWB by month 6, as in the case of auranofin, one might be tempted to say that a half-QALY had been added, at a cost of $12,500 (i.e. $300/.024), and that a full QALY could be costed at $25,000.

This would be erroneous, however. Auranofin did not add 2.4 per cent of full

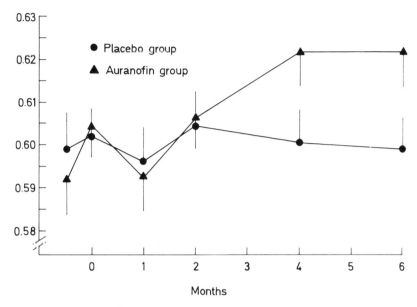

Figure 1. Scores on Quality of Well-Being Questionnaire.

health during the entire six months. As seen in Figure 1, the gain of 0.024 on the QWB was not reached until month 4. In fact apparently because of the slow onset of activity of auranofin, there was no significant QWB gain seen until after month 2. This was true for most of the measures in the trial, and was seen with the traditional measures in earlier auranofin trials. This delay presents an analytic problem, because in order to produce 2.4 per cent of a QALY the 0.024 gain on the QWB for months 4 and 6 would have to be experienced for a full year, that is in each of months 1 through 3, 4 through 6, and 7 through 12 as well. While the average QWB score during the first six months could be calculated fairly accurately from the data, it would be fundamentally wrong simply to assume it would be duplicated in the second six months, since the delayed onset of activity would not repeat itself. In fact only the level score from months 4 through 6 supports the assumption that there is no further improvement in months 7 through 12. Or there could be a worsening in these months. There would almost certainly be patients withdrawn from assigned medication and given a variety of treatments with unforseeable costs. Therefore, problems not clearly foreseen when the trial was replanned to encompass six months instead or twelve came to the fore when the cost-per-QALY analysis was attempted. Of course, none of this invalidates the other cost-effectiveness ratios discussed above. They must simply be understood as expressing the cost of *increasing* quality of life up to the amounts indicated, between the start and end of the trial.

The cost-per-QALY analysis underlines the fact that at best it would have been based on the first year of auranofin treatment. Only by chance would the second year have been similar. This raises the question of what period of treatment the cost-per-QALY analyses other therapies have been based on. This is important, because QALY measures, like cost-effectiveness measures generally, are relative: there is no way to know, except by comparison with ratios for other treatments, whether a ratio is high or low. Similarly, there is the basic issue of which control agent may have been used. In some analyses of other therapies, the alternative treatment may have been active, not placebo, and nearly as effective as the treatment in question. In other analyses, the alternative might have been to do nothing. Table 8 shows how this could affect the ratio for auranofin itself. In this table it is assumed that a full, typical year of data has been collected and that the QALY figure is based on an average 'steady state' over the entire twelve months. The top example shows a comparison with placebo, cumulating $1000 in costs over the twelve months (say for doctor visits and physiotherapy with $100 for inactive capsules) and producing a loss of 0.001 QALY for the period; this vs physiotherapy plus auranofin, costing $1,600 and producing a gain of 0.0023 QALYs. The cost-per-QALY ratio for auranofin is thus $600/0.024 QALY added or $25,000 per whole QALY. If, however, the comparison had been against no drug (visits and physiotherapy only at $900), quality of life with no drug might have been low and the contribution of auranofin relatively greater, giving a cost per added QALY of $17,500. Comparison against Agent X would give only $10,000 per QALY, but against Agent Y would give $60,000 per QALY. The problem of judging whatever ratio is produced for auranofin against ratios for therapies in other diseases would seem unmanageable if their ratios are similarly dependent on the alternative therapy. It would seem critical that the control treatment be that which in fact would always be employed were the study treatment not available. It is not always clear that such was the case when ratios for other therapies are presented.

Table 8. Hypothetical alternative $/QALY ratios

	Placebo	Auranofin	Added cost/Added QALY
(a)	$1,000/−0.001 −	$1,600/+0.23	= $600/0.024 = $25,000/1.000
(b)	No Drug	Auranofin	
	$ 900/−0.017 −	$1,600/+0.023	= $700/0.040 = $17,500/1.000
(c)	Agent X	Auranofin	
	$1,500/+0.013 −	$1,600/+0.023	= $100/0.010 = $10,000/1.000
(d)	Agent Y	Auranofin	
	$1,000/+0.013 −	$1,600/+0.023	= $600/0.010 = $60,000/1.000

Discussion

What conclusions might be drawn from the execution and analysis of this trial? An obvious one is that the many measures used and the uniform direction of their results, along with the high statistical significance of many of those results both singly and when grouped into composites, provide overwhelming evidence that auranofin improved quality of life. Rheumatologists familiar with traditional measures of disease process—joint counts, grip strength readings, walk time, and the like— and personally experienced with their correlation to patient reports of well-being might have inferred that changes in these convenient measures represent similar changes in quality of life. However, one may doubt whether other interested parties, including patients, would have come to this conclusion. Indeed when the trial was planned there was no strong consensus among the participating physicians that such an improvement would be quantified by the trial. Thus, the trial has provided evidence of an effect which the sceptic or the non-rheumatologist would most probably have overlooked when attempting to judge the therapeutic value of the compound.

The results of the trial tend to demystify the notion of quality of life. It would seem to be a robust enough thing, however fuzzily defined, to make itself known in a uniform way in a variety of contexts. It now appears quite possible to use plausible available instruments, both of the general-health and disease-specific type, as well as to construct simple global-impression scales, to detect an effect of therapy on broad relevant measures of health without worrying about whether quality of life has been correctly defined. Measures of daily function, as long as they are the result of systematic efforts to include major activities related to health, would seem more likely than not to be sensitive to treatment effect.

Results of the trial may help us to sort out which types of instrument provide the more meaningful measures of outcome. To attempt this, we might imagine that Drug A produced a treatment effect of $+16$ per cent of baseline standard deviation on Instrument X, aimed at functional ability, while an alternative but not identical Drug B produced the same effect of $+16$ per cent of baseline standard deviation on Instrument Y, also focused on functional ability. (As explained above, this method of expressing outcomes on differently calibrated measures in the same terms, i.e. percentage of baseline standard deviation, was that used in the trial to construct the composite measures of treatment effect.) We can further imagine that p-values are equal. Finally, we can imagine that both instruments are equally reliable, that is each gives identical results every time. If the results of the two instruments are the only information available, which drug should be selected for treatment? If Instrument X incorporates adverse effects and Instrument Y does not, Drug A would seem to be a better choice. This would argue for the QWB over the Keitel, Toronto, and HAQ. Similarly if Instrument X incorporates preferences and Y does not, Drug A would again be the better choice. Again this argues for the QWB. The whole notion of validity and its various types is relevant to the decision; but two essential aspects of validity in relation to quality-of-life measurement are clarified by this imaginary situation.

Similarly, if Instruments X and Y were of the simple global impression type, and if Instrument X specifically asked the patient to consider total health and adverse effects whereas Instrument Y was directed at arthritis activity, all else being equal, a +16 per cent on Instrument X should be more useful basis of drug selection than a +16 per cent on Instrument Y. Among the instruments in the trial, this would favour the Overall Health Ladder Scale over the Arthritis Ladder Scale, although adverse effects were not specifically mentioned in relation to the former. They probably should have been.

What if Instrument X were of the functional ability type, with adverse effects and preference weights incorporated, as in the QWB, and Instrument Y were the Overall Health Ladder Scale (or Overall Health 10-Centimetre line) with adverse effects mentioned for consideration? If they showed a +16 percent treatment effect for Drug A and B respectively, which drug should be favoured? It would seem that Drug A would be a better choice because the component items and weights of Instrument X give a rational, concrete explanation for the +16 per cent observed. There appears to be no way to test the validity of the global impression type measure except by its correlation to other measures for which validity as been tested in other ways. The same problem exists for the most statistically significant measured (p = 0.001) in the trial, the Arthritis Categorical Scale, scored simply 1 (worst) to 5, for categories from 'very poor' to 'very good'. Yet the 'how are you today' type question is one which some physicians have claimed is the most sensitive and useful, at least to them, when evaluating the quality-of-life changes in patients.

Finally, imagine that the QWB showed a +16 per cent for Drug A and the Patient Utility Measurement Set (PUMS) showed a +16 per cent for Drug B. Both incorporate adverse effects and patient preferences, the latter incorporating individual preferences fundamentally into each individual's score. The 100-point scale of the PUMS is not 'empty' of precise content as are the global impression scales and 10-centimetre lines, since a point along the PUMS continuum is determined by identified quantities of risk or sacrifice acceptable to the patient. Evaluating in depth the QWB and the PUMS is beyond the scope of this paper. Perhaps Pauker, McNeil and Torrance will address the relative merits of the two instruments when they report in detail on use of the PUMS in the trial.

It becomes clear that to be meaningful a quality-of-life instrument should further a judgement as to the practical importance of the score observed. The traditional measures do not do this, since their units of measure, such as millimetres of mercury or seconds of walk time, have little if any meaning in the context of daily life. For example, it is probably only those rheumatologists experienced in the use of traditional measures and the literature about them who would know how the grip strength of healthy 16 year-old boys, say, compares with that of 60 year-old women, let alone how grip strength may be expected to change with different therapies. The global measures' units have no bridge whatever to concrete experience, so that the therapeutic importance of a score change is unknowable by itself. Only through repeated correlation of the results with other concrete results can the global measures take on meaning. Of the simple, scalar type measures perhaps the 10-centimetre Pain Line comes closest to having built up a meaningful framework of such correlations. This argues for quality-of-life instruments with component items based on performance, since these have meaning in terms of common experience. Indeed, the score changes on the HAQ and QWB can be expressed in terms of change in performance of a single daily act, and the importance of the ability to perform that act or not can be reasonably judged. While the PUMS does not have performance items, its score appears amenable to the same kind of translation into experientially meaningful units—for example chances of death or years of life.

Unless concrete equivalents of the QWB or PUMS scores are eked out, the practical importance of a score change requires the same kind of framework of prior correlational experience that any other unfamiliar measure requires. That the two measures each employ a 100-point continuum and are each anchored by death and full health helps orient the lay evaluator but does not communicate the practical importance of, say, a +16 point change—even if expressed as percentage of full health. Theoretically, this need not detract from the value of these instruments. If the QWB or PUMS were used often enough, we should grasp the meaning a +16 degrees PUMS as readily as we do a +16 degrees Fahrenheit. It should be kept in mind, however, that the QWB requires carefully trained interviewers and twenty minutes of administration time. The PUMS requires the same if not more training effort, and a somewhat more lengthy but considerably more complex administration session.

The need, then, is for an instrument which includes adverse effects and patient preferences as comprehensively as does the QWB or the PUMS, which produces scores that speak more immediately to concrete experience and hence therapeutic importance, and which can be administered reliably with little or no training. As the QWB and PUMS are already such ingenious and cogent constructions, it is probably presumptuous to ask for simplicity as well. Nevertheless, the need is there.

The problems of cost-effectiveness evaluation in the context of a controlled clinicaltrial have been touched on above. On the one hand, the notion of an experimental control group is an appealing one to health economists, and clinical trials seem to offer opportunities that should not be missed. On the other hand, the very features which make for good science in the demonstration of efficacy— elimination of all possible causative variables other than the compound itself (such as patient non-compliance, particularly in the presence of adverse effects or the absence of therapeutic effect) and the imposition of whatever monitoring measures, no matter how frequent or invasive, are needed to document physiological changes—work directly against measurement of both effectiveness and cost. In fact, unless a clinical trial used in cost-effectiveness analysis is designed specifically for such purposes—in which case it may well not satisfy purists in efficacy determination—it should be suspect until shown useful. We can perhaps best appreciate this if we imagine an alternative, 'real world' experiment in which patients are randomized to either known auranofin or nothing (i.e. continuation of prior therapy), seen by their physician at whatever frequency is normal or appropriate in the individual situation, interviewed at home once a month about quality of life and events affecting cost, and then perhaps at month 6 given a complete medical examination. In contrast, the use of placebo in the actual trial stands out as an artificiality, one which would tend to reduce the residual efficacy (treatment effect) of auranofin. Use of a placebo could thus be described as a conservative or 'downside' scenario for cost-effectiveness purposes. The monthly visits required by the trial do not appear likely to have generated physician knowledge leading to new therapeutic manoeuvres, and the visit costs can be eliminated for the placebo group when the costs of the two groups are compared. Thus, the fact that the trial design was conservative and close to normal conditions of use allowed a relevant cost analysis to be undertaken. It is clear, however, how easily various artificialities typical of efficacy trials—for example, X-rays at month 4, with non-improved placebo patients switched to auranofin—might have confounded both effectiveness and cost determinations. Perhaps the best conclusion is that a cost-effectiveness evaluation should never be presumed to be possible in the context of a controlled clinical trial and, if thought possible, should not be undertaken lightly. Certainly, calculation of QALYs, especially in trials lasting less than a year, should be very carefully considered in advance.

Finally, when all is done, one is left with a ratio relating effectiveness, as expressed by a score, to cost. Ideally, the score will be in understandable quality-of-life units. Without that, judging whether a ratio is good or bad depends on comparison with ratios produced for other treatments in other studies. Certainly this is true when the unit of effectiveness is a QALY. Until a body of results is built up, perhaps the most meaningful way to relate effectiveness to cost is to proceed directly from the score to the expression of a specific daily task the average patient is able to do as a result of treatment. That improvement can then be judged in relation to its cost.

References

Anderson, J. P. and Moser, R. J. (1985). *Journal of the American Medical Association*, **253**, 2229–35.

Balaban, D. J., Sagi, P. C., Goldfarb, N. I. and Nettler, S. (1986). *Medical Care*, **24**, 973–80.

Bombardier, C. and Tugwell, P. (1983). *Journal of Rheumatology*, **10** (supplement), 68–73.

Bombardier, C., Ware, J., Russell, L. J., Larson, M., Chalmers, A. and Read, J. L. (1986). *American Journal of Medicine*, **81**, 565–76.

Brook, R. H., Ware, J. E. Davies-Avery, A. *et al.* (1979). *Medical Care*, **17** (supplement), 95–7.

Bush, J. W., Chen, M. and Patrick, D. L. (1973). Cost-effectiveness Using a Health Care Status Index. Analysis of the New York State PKU Screening Program. In *Health Care Status Indexes* ed. Berg, R. Chicago: Hospital Research and Educational Trust.

Dickson, J. S. and Bird, II. A. (1981). *Annals of Rheumatic Diseases*, **40**, 87–9.

Eberl, D. R., Fasching, V., Rahlfs, V., Schleyer, I. and Wolf, R. (1976). *Arthritis and Rheumatism*, **19**, 1278-86.

Fries, J. F., Spitz, P. W. and Young, D. Y. (1982). *Journal of Rheumatology*, **9**, 789–93.

Fries, J. F. (1985). Measurement of the Quality of Life: Development of the Health Assessment Questionnaire (HAQ). In *Rheumatology*, ed. Brooks, P. M. and York, J. R. New York: Elsevier.

Helewa, A., Goldsmith, C. H. and Smythe, H. A. (1982). *Journal of Rheumatology*, **9**, 794–7.

Husaini, B. A., Neff, J. A., Harrington, J. B., Hughes, M. D. and Stone, R. H. (1979). Depression in Rural Communities: Establishing CES-D Cutting Points. In *Mental Health Project, Final Report National Institute of Mental Health contract*, 278-77-0044 [DBE].

Kaplan, R. M., Bush, J. W. and Berry, C. C. (1976). *Health Services Research*, **11**, 478–507.

Kaplan, R. M., Bush, J. W. and Berry, C. C. (1978). The Reliability, Stability and Generalizability of a Health Status Index. In *Proceedings of the American Statistical Association, Social Statistics Section*, 704–9.

Melzack, R. (1975). *Pain*, **1**, 227–99.

Pauker, S. G., Torrance, G. W. and McNeil, B. J. (in preparation).

Radloff, L. S. (1977). *Applied Psychological Measurement*. **1**, 385–401.

Rosenshein, M. S., Farwell, V. T., Price, T. H., Larson, E. B. and Dale, D. C. (1980). *New England Journal of Medicine*, **302**, 1058–62.

Scott, J. and Huskisson, E. C. (1976). *Pain*, **2**, 175–84.

Thompson, M. S. (1986). *American Journal of Public Health*, **76**, 392–6.

Thompson, M. S. *Journal of Rheumatology*, forthcoming.

Measuring Health: A Practical Approach
Edited by G. Teeling Smith

9

Assessment of Treatment in Heart Disease

Bernie O'Brien

Health Economics Research Group, Brunel University, Uxbridge

Introduction

One in every three deaths in England and Wales in 1985 was due to Coronary Heart Disease (CHD). A total of 163,104 people had their lives cut short prematurely by the disease. Just over half of the victims were male and nearly a fifth were in the age group 45–64. Internationally, the countries of the UK occupy three of the top five places in the mortality rate league table with Northern Ireland experiencing a rate of 630 per thousand for males aged 40–69 years (Uemura and Pisa, 1985).

The burden of the disease is not limited to mortality. CHD accounted for 2.13 million bed-days in English hospitals in 1984 (Office of Population Censuses and Surveys, 1986) and some 814,000 people consult their General Practitioner (GP) during the year because of the disease (Royal College of General Practitioners, 1986). In terms of direct health service expenditures an estimated £390m (1985 prices) is attributable to CHD every year (Wells, 1987).

This growing burden of illness has been mirrored by medical and surgical advances in treatment for CHD. Interventions currently include medicines such as beta blockers for relief of angina, surgery such as coronary artery bypass grafting (CABG), the 'balloon catheter' principle of percutaneous translumial coronary angioplasty (PTCA), thrombolysis, pacemaker implantation, and the most radical surgical intervention of heart transplantation.

191

As the treatment possibilities and technology have advanced there has been a growing awareness of the need to evaluate new (and existing) modalities in terms of their resource costs and patient benefits. The need for treatment evaluation has arisen for two basic reasons. Firstly, as Cochrane (1972) has argued, there is a need to assess the effectiveness of new treatments relative to other modalities and/or placebo using the methodological framework of the Randomized Controlled Trial (RCT) before they are introduced into routine clinical practice. Secondly, for the purposes of resource allocation in the National Health Service (NHS) at a national and local level, it is desirable to know the relationship between effectiveness (benefit) *and* resource costs for treatment programmes that are competing for limited health care resources. The availability of such data would thus enable resource allocation priorities to be made which would produce the maximum effectiveness (patient benefit) from the available resources.

The extent to which progress can be made (particularly in the second area) depends largely upon a measurable definition of health being available. Although there are a variety of tests and measures for assessing the *clinical efficacy* of cardiac treatment (e.g. cardiac output and function), ultimately the effectiveness of treatment is quantified in terms of its beneficial impact on patient health. A simple representation of patient health is to consider it in two basic dimensions: changes in life-expectancy and changes in health-related quality of life such as the relief of anginal pain and restoration of other physical, social and emotional functioning.

The aim of this chapter is to focus on the measurement of health in the treatment of heart disease. In particular the assessment of quality of life, for which there are a growing number of measurement instruments available. The first section is a brief review of disease and health measurement instruments employed in studies of cardiac treatment ranging from simple return to work data to the use of the more sophisticated quality-of-life scales and instruments. In the second section data are presented from our recent economic evaluation of the UK heart transplant programmes (Buxton *et al.*, (1985). This case-study is not intended as a 'blueprint' for health benefit measurement but rather as a practical guide to the use of one available measure—the Nottingham Health Profile.

Health, Disease and Return to Work

There are a number of comprehensive guides to the conceptualization, definition and measurement of health, for example Culyer (1983), Teeling Smith (1985) and more recently Brooks (1986). There are three main observations which emerge from such literature:

1. Health is not merely the absence of disease but it extends to aspects of physical, social and emotional functioning.
2. Health is a multi-dimensional and value-laden concept.
3. There exists no simple or single 'gold standard' for measuring health.

The history of treatment evaluation in heart disease (and other areas) reflects these three factors. The traditional view of patient benefit finds origin in a disease-based medical model which relies heavily (often exclusively) on survival data. Yet to rely solely on life extension as the measure of benefit is implicitly to bias treatment comparisons against those modalities which generate qualitative changes (e.g. reductions in pain and disability) at the expense of survival. Evidence from McNeil *et al.* (1981) has indicated (not surprisingly) that patients are not indifferent about quality of life and are often willing to 'trade' life-expectancy for quality-of-life gains when choosing between treatments.

But the phrase 'quality of life' is a relatively recent addition to the vocabulary of treatment evaluation. The terminology used in a number of early cardiac treatment studies was that of patient 'rehabilitation' (for example, see Harris, 1970) following some intervention such as bypass surgery. The idea was to gauge the extent to which patients were being returned (or were achieving) a 'normal' healthy lifestyle following operation. Often a reliable indicator of such rehabilitation is the ability to return to work and such data are a common feature in many cardiac treatment evaluations (e.g. Barnes *et al.*, 1977; Ross *et al.*, 1978, 1981; Niles *et al.*, 1979; Love, 1980).

Return to work is a useful health indicator but has many limitations. Firstly, the ability to return to paid employment will be highly influenced by the nature of the job—is it possible to compare return to manual labour with return to a management job? Different occupations make different demands on physical, mental and social functioning: work capacity is therefore job-specific and not a universal indication of health status. Secondly, return to paid employment is a narrow definition which cannot be applied to those outside the labour force such as the elderly (where bypass surgery is becoming more common). In addition there is the question of unemployment—due allowance must be made for those who wish to return to paid employment but who cannot (for reasons other than their health) find a job. In summary therefore it is the *ability* to return to normal work activities, be they housework or paid employment, which is of interest as an indicator of normal functioning.

Such limitations of return-to-work data as a qualitative endpoint measure of rehabilitation have led investigators to attempt to scale and quantify those elements of physical, social and emotional functioning which comprise health status or quality of life. Such measures range from simple symptom scales or checklists to elaborate questionnaire-based health profiles and indices.

Disease Scales and Health Profiles

One of the earliest and still most widely used classification systems for heart disease patients is the New York Heart Association (NYHA) Classification. (New York Heart Association, 1964; Harris, 1970). The main element of the NYHA measure is four functional classes. Each class is differentiated by a descriptive scenario which combines elements of disease state, physical activity limitation, discomfort and symptoms. These classifications are presented in Table 1.

Table 1. New York Heart Association: functional classification

---

Class I:
   Patients with cardiac disease but without resulting limitations of physical activity. Ordinary physical activity does not cause undue fatigue, palpitation, dyspnoea, or anginal pain.

Class II:
   Patients with cardiac disease resulting in slight limitation of physical activity. They are comfortable at rest. Ordinary physical activity results in fatigue, palpitation, dyspnoea or anginal pain.

Class III:
   Patients with cardiac disease resulting in marked limitation of physical activity. They are comfortable at rest. Less than ordinary physical activity causes fatigue, palpitation, dyspnoea or anginal pain.

Class IV:
   Patients with cardiac disease resulting in inability to carry on any physical activity without discomfort. Symptoms of cardiac insufficiency or of anginal syndrome may be present even at rest. If any physical activity is undertaken, discomfort is increased.

Source: New York Heart Association (1964).

The NYHA system is widely reported in the cardiac literature for assessing functional change: Weinstein *et al.* (1981); Guyatt *et al.* (1985); Pennock *et al.* (1983). An example of NYHA classes being used as an indicator of patient outcome is the reporting of results from the Stanford heart transplant programme by Pennock *et al.* (1982). They note that pre-transplant the vast majority of candidates were in NYHA Class IV and that of the 106 survivors at 1 year post-transplant, 97 per cent were in NYHA Class I functional status. (Similar alternatives to NYHA include the Canadian Cardiovascular Society classifications used in the Coronary Artery Surgery Study (CASS, 1983) and the Specific Activity Scale (SAS) reported in Goldman *et al.* (1981).)

Another common classification of functional status is the Karnofsky Index which was originally developed for the evaluation of chemotherapy as a treatment for cancer (Karnofsky and Burchenal, 1949). The measure has gained wider application such as assessment of function in renal dialysis (Gutman *et al.*, 1981) and more recently in the US evaluation of heart transplantation (Evans *et al.*, 1984).

The Karnofsky Index is a simple scale form 1 to 10 and patients are assigned to categories by a clinician or other health care professional. To illustrate the use of the Karnofsky Index in heart disease treatment, data from the US National Heart Transplantation Study are presented in Table 2. These data indicate a marked shift in the distribution of patient classification before and after transplant. Thus following heart transplantation 66.3 per cent of recipients were judged to be 'normal' with no complaints or evidence of disease, whereas prior to transplantation 23.6 per cent of patients were 'very sick' and requiring hospitalization.

Table 2. Functional impairment before and after heart transplantation (Karnofsky Index)

		Percentage of patients	
		Before	After
1.	Normal: no complaints: no evidence of disease	0.2	66.3
2.	Able to carry on annual activity: minor signs and symptoms of disease	0.0	23.2
3.	Normal activity with effort: some signs and symptoms of disease	0.0	6.1
4.	Cares for self: unable to carry on normal activity or do active work	3.1	0.6
5.	Requires occasional assistance but is able to care for most of own needs	6.2	2.8
6.	Requires considerable assistance and requent medical care	13.1	1.1
7.	Disabled: requires special care and assistance	31.2	0.0
8.	Severely disabled: hospitalization is indicated although death not imminent	12.6	0.0
9.	Very sick: hospitalization necessary	23.6	0.0
10.	Moribund: fatal processes progressing rapidly	9.3	0.0

Source. Evans *et al.* (1984): Tables 21-E-5, 25–5.

There are two criticisms that can be made of measurement instruments such as NYHA and Karnofsky. The first is that they are a categorization of patients by a doctor or other health professional and are therefore clinical judgements concerning disease state. This is not a criticism *per se* only to the extent that such judgements differ from results obtained by patient *self-rating* functional measures. In the Evans *et al.* (1984) study of heart transplantation, for example, there was a wide discrepancy between patients' self-rating of post-transplant function as measured by the Sickness Impact Profile (SIP) (Bergner *et al.*, 1981) and the clinician's rating of patients on the Karnofsky Index, with the latter rating patients as being less impaired than the former.

The second criticism is that a measure such as Karnofsky is often reported as a mean 'score' ranging between 0 and 10 for a group of patients. Yet there is no reason to suppose that the intervals between the ten categories represent the same degree of dysfunction. Often it is implicitly assumed that the scale is a simple linear ratio scale and that a move from category 2 to 3 is as 'bad' (in terms of disability or dysfunction) as a move from 8 to 9. Yagi and Crowley (1984), for example, in the survival analysis of heart transplantation use pre-transplantation Karnofsky 'scores' as a linear covariate in a proportional hazards model to predict post-transplant survival. But to move towards a true interval or ratio scale what is required is some indication of the relative importance or severity of differing degrees of disability or pain, etc. associated with each disease state or clinical classification. To achieve such calibration, judgements must be made and the values of patients and the public invoked. The definition (and measurement) of health therefore broadens from medical science with the emphasis on disease scales to include aspects of social science with its emphasis on the measurement of values and elicitation of preferences concerning the various components of health status.

A number of social scientists have therefore worked with clinicians to construct questionnaire-based instruments for assessing quality of life which reflect patients' own perceptions of their health state in its various dimensions. The construction of such instruments has employed the use of a variety of scaling techniques such that health profiles or indices are interval or ratio scales, rather than simple nominal or ordinal scales. The relative valuations for scaling health dimensions (e.g. degrees of physical functioning, pain, etc.) are typically derived from random samples of the general population who are asked (in various ways) to rate the relative importance or value to them of differing levels of impairment, pain, distress, etc.

In Table 3, six of the most widely-used and well-validated instruments for assessing health are presented. This table is taken from the review by Wenger *et al* (1984) of the measurement of quality-of-life in cardiovascular clinical trials. As can be seen from Table 3 the length, administration-time and method of administration vary widely with the SIP containing 136 items and a completion time of 30 minutes, down to Psychological General Well-Being Index (22 items and 12 minutes). The most complex to administer is the Quality of Well-Being Scale (QWB) which requires a trained interviewer. An important practical point to note when selecting an appropriate instrument for evaluative research is whether postal follow-up of patients and self-completion is required in which case QWB would be inappropriate and compliance may suffer with some of the lengthier self-completion scales such as SIP.

Table 3. Six instruments for measuring health

Instrument	Dimensions examined	Length	Administration (time in minutes)
Sickness Impact Profile (Bergner et al., 1981)	Physical: ambulation, mobility, body care Psychosocial: social interaction, communication, alertness, emotional behaviour Other: sleep/rest, eating, work/home management, recreational pastimes	136 items	Self or interviewer (30')
McMaster Health Index Questionnaire (Chambers et al., 1982)	Physical: mobility, self-care, communication and global physical functioning Social: general well-being, work/social role performance, social support and participation and global social function Emotional: self-esteem, findings about personal relationships and the future, critical life events, and global emotional functioning	59 items	Self-administered (20')
Nottingham Health Profile (Hunt et al., 1981)	Six domains of experience: pain, physical mobility, sleep, emotional reactions, energy, social isolation Seven domains of daily life: employment, household work, relationships, personal life, sex, hobbies, vacations	45 items	Self-administered (10')
Psychological General Well-Being Index (Fazio, 1977)	Six dimensions: freedom from bodily distress, life satisfaction, sense of vitality, cheerful vs distressed, relaxed vs anxious, self-control	22 items	Self or interviewer (12')
General Health Rating Index (Ware et al., 1978)	Six dimensions: past, present, and future perceptions of health; health-related worry and concern; resistance vs susceptibility to illness; tendency to view illness as a part of life	29 items	Self or interviewer (7')
Quality of Well-Being Scale (Bush, 1984)	Measures actual performance and preference; self-care, mobility, institutionalization, social activities, reports of symptoms and problems, including mental	50 items	Trained interviewer (12')

Source: Wenger et al. (1984).

SIP is probably the most widely used of all of the instruments listed, and in the area of cardiac treatment it has been used in the US heart transplantation evaluation study (Evans *et al.*, 1984) and also in the assessment of cardiac arrest and myocardial infarction patients (Bergner *et al.*, 1985). In this latter study, 308 cardiac arrest patients were age- and sex-matched with myocardial infarction controls and both groups were interviewed six months following the cardiac event. SIP scores for the two groups are presented in Table 4.

Table 4. SIP scores for matched pairs of survivors of cardiac arrest and myocardial infarction (N = 308)

Category	Cardiac arrest Mean		Myocardial infarction Mean	
Sleep and rest	14.2		11.5	
Emotional behaviour	8.2		6.1	
Body care and movement	4.1		2.4	
Household management	17.3		12.1	
Mobility	8.4		4.2	
Social interaction	9.8		6.3	
Ambulation	10.7		7.7	
Alertness	11.7		6.5	
Communication	5.4		2.9	
Work	27.1		17.0	
Recreation and pastimes	19.7		15.2	
Eating behaviour	6.5		6.8	
Physical	6.9	(11.2)	4.0	(6.5)
Psychosocial	8.8	(1.24)	5.6	(9.5)
Total SIP	10.3	(10.8)	6.9	(7.8)

Source: Bergner *et al.* (1985).
Note: ( ) denotes standard deviation.

A mean score for each category of SIP can be calculated and also a total SIP score with a range of 0 to 100, where a higher score indicates a poorer health status. In addition the categories can be aggregated in such a way as to produce a total 'physical' score and a 'psychosocial' score. The Bergner study therefore suggests that survivors of cardiac arrest had a marginally higher level of dysfunction than that observed in infarction controls; this observation holding true for total SIP scores as well as both component dimensions of physical and psychosocial dysfunction.

Health Indices and Utility Measurement

If the composite measure of health is quantity as well as quality of life, the health profile approach does not resolve the issue of how these two elements can be aggregated into a single quantum. The concept of Quality Adjusted Life Years (QALYs) as a composite health outcome measure was formalized by Weinstein and Stason (1977) although the idea had previously been used by Klarman *et al.* (1968) in his study of renal transplantation vs dialysis. In Klarman's study, for example, he argued that a year of survival with dialysis was equivalent to 75 per cent of a year with a functioning graft. The simple idea therefore is that when comparing two treatment regimes in terms of life-year gains, the quality of those life-year gains (e.g. are they disability- or pain-free years?) is incorporated as an 'adjustment' factor to life-expectancy.

There exist a variety of methods for quality-adjusting life-years which range in complexity. At a simple level freedom from symptoms, NYHA class or degree of angina (mild/moderate/severe) might be used as the adjustment factor for survival on a given regime. As discussed earlier, however, these ratings and adjustments are undertaken by an external observer rather than being a patient self-rating. Yet even if a self-rating profile measure such as SIP is used there still exist no preference data on the trade-offs between quantity and quality of life and hence no sound basis for combining SIP data with life-expectancy to construct QALYs.

An alternative approach is to construct a health or utility index which rates health states relative to each other and to death. There are a number of scaling techniques for constructing such a measure. Torrance (1986) provides an excellent survey of health utility measurement which includes both the *standard gamble* approach and the *Time Trade-off* approach which is explained and illustrated by Buxton in this volume (Chapter 5). Both of these methods are *implicit* scaling methods because they impute valuations indirectly from hypothetical choices. An *explicit* scaling approach was devised by Rosser and Watts (1972) (see also Williams, Chapter 11 this volume) to construct a health index which has been used by Williams (1986) to quality-adjust life-expectancy gains in his study of the cost-effectiveness of coronary bypass surgery relative to medical management.

In summary, there are a growing number of instruments available for assessing quality-of-life changes in cardiac and other treatment areas. In particular, health profiles such as SIP have been applied in a wide variety of study contexts. In the next part of this chapter we go on to describe in more detail the content and application of one such profile instrument—the Nottingham Health Profile.

Heart Transplantation: A Case-study

In this section data are presented from our recent economic evaluation of the heart transplant programmes at Harefield and Papworth hospitals. A full account of costs and benefit measurement can be found in Buxton *et al.* (1985) and the relationship between survival gains and quality of life is further explained in O'Brien *et al.* (1987).

In the absence of a rigorous experimental study design such as a Randomized Controlled Trial (RCT) it was difficult to determine the extent to which transplantation was life-extending for recipients. However, the available evidence suggested that there were gains in life-years. Therefore, the second strand of patient benefit measurement was to assess qualitative changes in the patient's life associated with the procedure. The following discussion is of our practical experience with the Nottingham Health Profile (NHP) in this assessment.

A number of early commentators had indicated that heart transplantation produces significant improvements in the recipient's quality of life. In an account of the early stages of the programme at Papworth hospital, English *et al*. (1982) state that 'the quality-of-life of the 14 survivors' who at the time of writing had been discharged from hospital 'has greatly improved, and most of the heart recipients are delighted with the degree of rehabilitation they have attained'. Similar reports from Stanford University have emphasized the importance of survivors' quality of life 'defined simply as restoration of overall functional capacity sufficient to provide the patient with an unrestricted option to return to active employment in an activity of choice' (Pennock *et al*., 1982).

Our UK study sought to answer two basic questions regarding patient quality of life:

1. Is transplantation associated with a significant and sustained improvement in the recipient's quality of life?
2. Following transplantation how does recipient quality of life compare with a normal 'healthy' population?

It was decided to limit our choice of measure to existing validated instruments that would require no additional development for use on heart transplant patients, thus enabling prospective data collection to begin as soon as possible. The added advantage of using an existing and widely used instrument was that NHP response data were available from a wide variety of studies and populations thus a range of possible comparison groups for our heart transplant data. Furthermore, it was decided that the measure should be a subjective health assessment by the patient, quite independent of clinical views. perceptions or expectations of prognosis.

A number of measures for assessing health were reviewed by our research team. These included the Index of Well-Being (IWB) (Bush *et al*., 1975) and the Sickness Impact Profile (SIP) (Bergner *et al*., 1981) which has been 'anglicized' by Patrick (1980) into the Functional Limitations Profile. In addition to these US-developed measures the Nottingham Health Profile (NHP) was considered—being a widely tested and utilized questionnaire measure of individuals' subjective perceptions of their health state (Hunt *et al*., 1986).

The NHP was chosen for a number of reasons:

i. it is sensitive to a wide range of health states;
ii. comparison population NHP responses were available;
iii. it can be administered by interview or mail;
iv. it makes relatively small demands on patient time and effort (an important factor given the pre-transplant morbid state).

The latter two points were seen as particularly important if we were to obtain repeated observations over time on the same patients.

Content and Structure of the NHP

The NHP was devised by a team from the Department of Community Health at Nottingham University School of Medicine (Hunt *et al.*, 1986). The profile consists of two parts. Part I sets out to measure subjective health status by asking for yes/no patient responses to a carefully selected set of 38 simple statements relating to six dimensions of social functioning: energy, pain, emotional reactions, sleep, social isolation and physical mobility. The actual statements that form each dimension and the weights applied to them are presented in Table 5 (see Appendix A for the questionnaire format). Respondents are required to answer 'yes' or 'no' to each statement. All statements relate to limitations on activity or aspects of 'distress'. All statements *in any given dimension* are weighted relative to each other; the range of possible scores in any dimension is 0–100. Dimension scores of 100 indicate the presence of all limitations listed, and a zero score the absence of limitations, but these two extreme dimension scores do not indicate death or 'perfect health'.

Part II of the Profile relates to seven areas of task performance affected by health (see Appendix A): occupation, ability to perform tasks around the home, personal relationships, sex life, social life, hobbies and holidays. Respondents answer 'yes' if their present state of health is causing problems with the particular activity. Part II has no weights; a simple count of affirmative responses is used as a summary statistic. These data are of more limited use than those from Part I and are not reported here.

Using the NHP

To provide quantitative estimates of health status differences between individuals and over time, patients completed the NHP at regular intervals before and after transplantation. In addition, a number of semi-structured interviews were undertaken with transplant candidates and recipients in order to investigate particular aspects of health and lifestyle in more detail.

Table 5. Nottingham health profile. Section 1: listing of statements and associated weights

Energy	
I soon run out of energy	24.00
Everything is an effort	36.80
I'm tired all of the time	39.20
	100.0
Pain	
I'm in pain when going up and down stairs or steps	5.83
I'm in pain when I'm standing	8.96
I find it painful to change position	9.99
I'm in pain when I'm sitting	10.49
I'm in pain when I walk	11.22
I have pain at night	12.91
I have unbearable pain	19.74
I'm in constant pain	20.86
	100.0
Emotional reactions	
The days seem to drag	7.08
I'm feeling on edge	7.22
I've forgotten what its like to enjoy myself	9.31
I lose my temper easily these days	9.76
Things are getting me down	10.47
I wake up feeling depressed	12.01
Worry is keeping me awake at night	13.95
I feel as if I'm losing control	13.99
I feel that life is not worth living	16.21
	100.0
Sleep	
I'm waking up in the early hours of the morning	12.57
It takes me a long time to get to sleep	16.10
I sleep badly at night	21.70
I take tablets to help me sleep	23.37
I lie awake for most of the night	27.26
	100.0
Social isolation	
I'm finding it hard to get on with people	15.97
I'm finding it hard to make contact with people	19.36
I feel there is nobody I am close to	20.13
I feel lonely	22.01
I feel I am a burden to people	22.53
	100.0
Physical mobility	
I find it hard to reach for things	9.30
I find it hard to bend	10.57
I have trouble getting up and down stairs and steps	10.79
I find it hard to stand for long (e.g. at the kitchen sink, waiting for a bus)	11.20
I can only walk about indoors	11.54
I find it hard to dress myself	12.61
I need help to walk about outside (e.g. walking aid or someone to support me)	12.69
I'm unable to walk at all	21.30
	100.0

Our aim was to use the NHP to provide information in four main areas:

1. Paired 'before and after' transplant profiles for individual patients would permit estimation of change in health state as a result of (or at least coincident with) transplant.
2. Monitoring NHP scores of patients accepted for, but prior to, transplantation would help to identify quality-of-life changes for transplant candidates following assessment.
3. Comparison of post-transplant NHP scores with existing data from a 'healthy' population would help to determine the extent to which transplant recipients achieved a 'normal' quality of life following the operation.
4. Monitoring Profile scores at regular intervals post-transplant would help to detect any longer term deterioration or improvement in quality of life.

In summary, potential candidates were identified at assessment where the questionnaire was administered by an interviewer in addition to a wide-ranging semi-structured interview concerning the impact of their health status on areas such as work and social life. For patients accepted onto the programme, the NHP was then completed at three-monthly intervals. For those transplanted the profile was then administered at three months following transplant, and then completed every three months as a postal follow-up.

Results

Given that the NHP scores are not 'true' numbers but are obtained from a scaling technique the appropriate statistical tests for testing hypotheses are non-parametric. A number of standard statistical computer packages such as BMDP (Dixon, 1983) are available for performing the relevant non-parametric tests.

A useful preliminary to formal analysis, however, is graphical inspection of the data. Figure 1 presents mean dimension scores as histograms over time from assessment to periods post-transplant. These observations are calculated from all 1,036 completed profiles that were available for analysis. The impression gained from Figure 1 is one of rapidly decreasing health status prior to transplant followed by a sharp improvement post-transplant which appears to be maintained thereafter.

There were 62 patients with 'pairs' of 'before and after' profiles and statistical comparison using the Wilcoxon test indicated significant ($p < 0.01$) improvement in all six dimensions of the profile. A number of statistical tests were performed to detect any change in NHP responses over time. There was some evidence of an increase in social isolation prior to transplant, but for all other dimensions, both before and after transplant, no significant trends were found in NHP responses. Hence the improvement following transplant appears to be a once-and-for-all shift in quality of life.

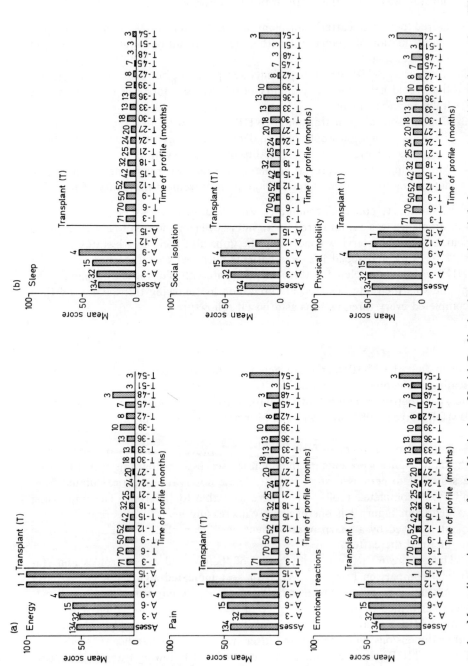

Figure 1. Mean dimension scores for the Nottingham Health Profile, by three month periods from assessment (A) and transplant (T) (number of observations above bars)

'Normal' population NHP response data were available from a random sample from Nottingham (Hunt *et al.*, 1984), and in the relevant age groups post- transplant scores were very similar to those observed in the population. Furthermore, it should be noted that 'normal' populations do not necessarily score zero on NHP dimensions; at any given point in time the population at large will have degrees of morbidity which constitute restrictions in their quality of life.

An important finding was that the NHP seemed to accord well with clinical judgement and patient classifications on the basis of morbidity and prognosis. An example of this was at Papworth where there exist two categories of transplant candidate—those who are *definitely* accepted and those who are *provisionally* accepted. The distinction is a clinical judgement based on prognosis; in crude terms the 'sicker' the patient the more likely they are to be definite candidates whereas the provisional candidates are thought able to wait for a longer period.

Applying the NHP to both patient groups we found that in all six dimensions of the NHP the 'definite' candidates were significantly worse ($P < 0.05$; Mann–Whitney test) than the 'provisional' candidates. This strong correlation with clinical judgement was useful in terms of demonstrating to clinicians the discriminatory power of the profile and was useful 'corroborative' support for the profile as an indicator of health status.

In summary, the NHP was a useful instrument for assessing quality-of-life in heart transplant patients. Its main advantages are that it has relatively few items, is easy to complete and analyse, and appears to correlate well with clinical judgements concerning differential patient health status.

Concluding Remarks

There is a wide variety of instruments available for the assessment of health outcomes following treatment for heart disease. They range in complexity from simple return to work data, symptom or disease scales, to health profiles, health indices and utility measurement methods. The question of which method is appropriate for a particular evaluation will depend upon the question being asked. In some contexts it may be more appropriate to use disease-specific measures (Guyatt *et al.*, 1986) which are sensitive to small but clinically significant changes. In other contexts the global quality-of-life measures (such as SIP or NHP) may be more appropriate.

Perhaps the ideal is to use a number of measures rather than to depend on the reliability of one instrument. The use of multiple instrument assessment also permits the investigators to combine the strengths and weaknesses of a range of methods which may target different areas of quality-of-life. Recent examples of multiple-instrument assessment include the multicentre clinical trial of captopril, methyldopa and propanolol (Croog *et al.*, 1986) and the study of oral gold (Auranofin) in the treatment of rheumatoid arthritis (Bombardier *et al.*, 1986). In the final analysis, however, such studies may be costly to perform and the practical reality of such evaluative research is that the additional benefits achieved by using multiple quality-of-life instruments must be balanced against the additional research costs which fall on the investigators and the patients.

References

Barnes, G. K., Ray, M. J., Oberman, A. *et al.* (1977). Changes in working status of patients following coronary bypass surgery. *Journal of the American Medical Association*, **238**(12), 1259–62.

Bergner, L., Hallstrom, A.P., Bergner, M. *et al.* (1985). Health status of survivors of cardiac arrest and of myocardial infarction controls, *American Journal of Public Health*, **75**, 1321–23.

Bergner, M., Bobbitt, R. A., Carter, W. B. and Gilson, B. S. (1981). The Sickness Impact Profile: development and final revision of a health status measure. *Medical Care*, **19**, 787–805.

Bombardier, C., Ware, J., Russell, I. J. *et al.* (1986). Auranofin therapy and quality of life in patients with rheumatoid arthritis. *American Journal of Medicine*, **81**(4), 565–77.

Brooks, R. G. (1986) *The Development and Construction of Health Status Measures*, Lund, Sweden: Institute of Health Economics.

Bush, J. W. (1984). General health policy model/ Quality of Well-Being (QWB) Scale. In Wenger, N. K. *et al.* (eds), *Assessment of Quality of Life in Trials of Cardiovascular Therapies*, New York: Le Jacq Publishing.

Bush, J. W., Blischke, W. R. and Berry, C. C. (1975). Health Indices, outcomes and the quality of medical care. In Yaffe, R. and Zalkind, D. (eds), *Evaluation in Health Services Delivery*, New York: Engineering Foundation.

Buxton, M. J., Acheson, R., Caine, N., Gibson, S. and O'Brien, B. J. (1985). *Costs and Benefits of the Heart Transplant Programmes at Harefield and Papworth Hospitals*, DHSS Research Report No. 12, London: HMSO.

CASS Principal Investigators and Their Associates (1983). Coronary Artery Surgery Study (CASS): A randomised trial of coronary artery bypass surgery. Quality of life in patients randomly assigned to treatment groups. *Circulation*, **68**, 951–60.

Chambers, L. W., MacDonald, L. A., Tugwell, P. *et al.* (1982). The McMaster Health Index Questionnaire as a measure of quality of life for patients with rheumatoid disease. *Journal of Rheumatology*, **9**, 780–4.

Cochrane, A. L. (1972). *Effectiveness and Efficiency: Random Reflections on Health Services*, London: Nuffield Provincial Hospital Trust.

Croog, S. H., Levine, S., Testa, M. A. *et al.* (1986). The effects of antihypertensive therapy on the quality of life. *New England Journal of Medicine*, **314**(26), 1657–64.

Culyer, A. J. (ed.) (1983). *Health Indicators*, Martin Robertson.

Dixon, W. J. (ed.) (1985). *BMDP Statistical Software*, 1985 Printing. Berkeley: University of California Press.

English, T. A. H., Cory-Pearce, R. and McGregor, C. (1982). Heart transplantation at Papworth Hospital. *Heart Transplantation*, **1**, 110–11.

Evans, R. W., Manninen, D. L., Overcast, T. D. *et al.* (1984). *The National Heart Transplantation Study: Final Report*, Seattle, Washington: Battelle Human Affairs Research Center.

Fazio, A. F. (1977). A concurrent validational study of the NCHS General Well-Being Schedule. *Vital and Health Statistics*, Series 2, no. 73. National Center for Health Statistics, Hyattsville, MD. DHEW Publ. No. (HRA) 78–1347.

Goldman, L., Hashimoto, D. and Cook, E. F. (1981). Comparative reproducibility and validity of systems for assessing cardiovascular functional class: advantages of a new Specific Activity Scale, *Circulation*, **64**, 1227–34.

Gutman, R. A., Stead, W. W., Robinson, R. R., (1981). Physical activity and employment status of patients on maintenance dialysis. *New England Journal of Medicine*, **304**, 309–13.

Guyatt, G. H., Bombardier, C., and Tugwell, P. X. (1986). Measuring disease-specific quality of life in clinical trials. *Canadian Medical Association Journal*, **314**, 889–95.

Guyatt, G. H., Thompson, P. J., Berman, L. B. *et al*. (1985). How should we measure function in patients with chronic heart and lung disease? *Journal of Chronic Diseases*, **38**(6), 517–24.

Hampton, J. R., (1984). Coronary artery bypass grafting for the reduction of mortality: an analysis of the trials. *British Medical Journal*, **289**, 1166–70.

Harris, R. (1970). Assessing the cardiac patient for rehabilitation. *New York State Journal of Medicine*, **70**, 511–15

Hunt, S. M., McEwen, J. and McKenna, S. P. (1986). *Measuring Health Status*, Beckenham, Kent: Croom Helm.

Hunt, S. M., McEwan, J. and McKenna, S. P. (1984). Perceived health: age and sex comparisons in a community. *Journal of Epidemiology and Community Health*, **38**, 156–60.

Hunt, S. M., McKenna, S. P., McEwan, J. *et al*. 1981. A quantitative approach to perceived health status: a validation study. *Journal of Epidemiology and Community Health*, **34**, 281–6.

Karnofsky, D. A. and Burchenal, J. H., (1949). The clinical evaluation of chemotherapeutic agents in cancer. In Macleod, C. M. (ed.), *Evaluation of Chemotherapeutic Agents*, New York, NY: Columbia University Press.

Klarman, H. E., Francis, J. and Rosenthal, G. D. (1968). Cost-effectiveness analysis applied to the treatment of chronic renal disease, *Medical Care*, **6**(48).

Love, J. W., (1980). Employment status after coronary bypass operations and some cost considerations, *Journal of Cardiovascular Surgery*, **80**, 68–72.

McNeil, B. J., Wechselbaum, R. and Pauker, S. G. (1981). Speech and survival: tradeoffs between quality and quantity of life in laryngeal cancer, *New England Journal of Medicine*, **305**, 982–7.

New York Heart Association (1964). *Diseases of the Heart and Blood Vessels: Nomenclature and Criteria for Diagnoses*, Boston: Little, Brown.

Niles, N. W., Vander Salm, T. J. and Cutler, B. S. (1979). Return to work after coronary artery bypass operation. *Journal of Cardiovascular Surgery*, **79**, 916–21.

O'Brien, B. J., Buxton, M. J. and Ferguson, B. (1987). Measuring the effectiveness of heart transplant programmes: quality of life data and their relationship to survival analysis. *Journal of Chronic Diseases*, **40**, suppl 1, 137–53.

Office of Population Censuses and Surveys (1986). *Hospital Inpatient Enquiry*, London: HMSO.

Patrick, D. (1980). Standardisation of comparative health status measures: using scales developed in America in an English speaking country! *Proc. Third Biennial Conference on Health Survey Research Methods*, National Center for Health Services Research.

Pennock, J. L., Reitz, B. A., Bieber, C. P. and Stinson, E. B. (1982). Cardiac transplantation in perspective for the future: survival, complications, rehabilitation and cost. *Journal of Cardiovascular Surgery*, **83**, 168–77.

Ross, J. K., Diwell, A. E., Marsh, J. L. *et al*. (1978). Wessex cardiac surgery follow-up survey: the quality of life after operation. *Thorax*, **33**, 3–9.

Ross, J. K., Monro, J. L., Diwell, A. E. *et al*. (1981). The quality of life after cardiac surgery. *British Medical Journal*, **272**, 451–3.

Rosser, R. M. and Watts. V. C. (1972). The measurement of hospital output. *International Journal of Epidemiology*, **1**, 361–7.

Royal College of General Practitioners (1986). *Third National Morbidity Survey*, London: HMSO.

Teeling-Smith, G. (1985). *Measurement of Health*, London: Office of Health Economics.

Torrance, G. W. (1986). Measurement of health state utilities for economic appraisal. *Journal of Health Economics*, **5**, 1–30.

Uemara, K. and Pisa, Z. (1985). *World Health Statistics Quarterly*, **38**, 142–62.

Ware, J. E., Davies-Avery, A. and Donald, C. A. (1978). *Conceptualization and Measurement of Health for Adults in the Health Insurance Study: Volume V, General Health Perceptions*. R-1981/5-HEW, Santa Monica: Rand Corporation.

Weinstein, M. C., Pliskin, J. S. and Stason, W. B. (1981). Coronary artery bypass surgery: decision and policy analysis. In Bunker, J. P. Barnes, B. A. and Mosteller, F. (eds) (1981), *Costs, Risks, and Benefits of Surgery*, New York: Oxford University Press.

Weinstein, M. C. and Stason, W. B. (1977). Foundations of cost effectiveness analysis for health and medical practices. *New England Journal of Medicine*, **296**, 716–21.

Wenger, N. K. *et al*, (1984). *Assessment of Quality of Life of Trials of Cardiovascular Therapies*, New York: Le Jacq Publishing.

Wells, N. E. J. (1987). *Coronary Heart Disease: the need for action*, London: Office of Health Economics.

Williams, A. (1986). Economics of coronary artery bypass grafting. *British Medical Journal*, **291**, 326–9.

Yagi, J. and Crowley, J. (1984). Survival of heart transplant Recipients. Chapter 21, in Evans, R. *et al*., *The National Heart Transplantation Study*.

Appendix A: The Nottingham Health Profile

Part I

Listed below are some problems people may have in their daily life.
Look down the list and put a tick in the box under **Yes** for any problem you have at the moment.
Tick the box **No** for any problem you do not have.

Please answer every question. If you are not sure whether to say yes or no, tick whichever answer you think is **more true** at the moment.

	Yes	No
I'm tired all the time	☐	☐
I have pain at night	☐	☐
Things are getting me down	☐	☐

	Yes	No
I have unbearable pain	☐	☐
I take tablets to help me sleep	☐	☐
I've forgotten what it's like to enjoy myself	☐	☐

	Yes	No
I'm feeling on edge	☐	☐
I find it painful to change position	☐	☐
I feel lonely	☐	☐

	Yes	No
I can only walk about indoors	☐	☐
I find it hard to bend	☐	☐
Everything is an effort	☐	☐

	Yes	No
I'm waking up in the early hours of the morning	☐	☐
I'm unable to walk at all	☐	☐
I'm finding it hard to make contact with people	☐	☐

	Yes	No
The days seem to drag	☐	☐
I have trouble getting up and down stairs or steps	☐	☐
I find it hard to reach for things	☐	☐

	Yes	No
I'm in pain when I walk	☐	☐
I lose my temper easily these days	☐	☐
I feel there is nobody I am close to	☐	☐

	Yes	No
I lie awake for most of the night	☐	☐
I feel as if I'm losing control	☐	☐
I'm in pain when I'm standing	☐	☐

	Yes	No
I find it hard to dress myself	☐	☐
I soon run out of energy	☐	☐
I find it hard to stand for long (eg. at the kitchen sink, waiting for a bus)	☐	☐

	Yes	No
I'm in constant pain	☐	☐
It takes me a long time to get to sleep	☐	☐
I feel I am a burden to people	☐	☐

	Yes	No
Worry is keeping me awake at night	☐	☐
I feel that life is not worth living	☐	☐
I sleep badly at night	☐	☐

	Yes	No
I'm finding it hard to get on with people	☐	☐
I need help to walk about outside (eg. a walking aid or someone to support me)	☐	☐
I'm in pain when going up and down stairs or steps	☐	☐

	Yes	No
I wake up feeling depressed	☐	☐
I'm in pain when I'm sitting	☐	☐

Part II

Now we would like you to think about the activities in your life which may be affected by health problems. In the list below, tick **Yes** for each activity in your life which is being affected by your state of health. Tick **No** for each activity which is not being affected, or which does not apply to you.

Is your present state of health causing problems with your ...

	Yes	No		Yes	No
Job of work (That is, paid employment)	□	□	Sex life	□	□
Looking after the home (Examples: cleaning and cooking, repairs, odd jobs around the home etc.)	□	□	Interests and hobbies (Examples: sports, arts and crafts, do-it-yourself etc.)	□	□
Social life (Examples: going out, seeing friends, going to the pub, etc.)	□	□	Holidays (Examples: summer or winter holidays, weekends away, etc.)	□	□
Home life (That is: relationships with other people in your home)	□	□			

10

Assessment of Treatment of Irritable Bowel Syndrome

Jane Stevens
Welsh School of Pharmacy, Cardiff
and
Centre for Medicines Research, Carshalton

Jeffrey Poston
Welsh School of Pharmacy, Cardiff

and

Stuart Walker
Centre for Medicines Research, Carshalton

Irritable Bowel Syndrome—The Disease

Irritable bowel syndrome is very common, accounting for almost half of the referrals to gastroenterologists (Heaton, 1983). It is characterized by abnormal gastro-intestinal transit which results in irregular bowel habits, often with underlying emotional disturbances (Crean *et al.*, 1984). Patients can experience one of two distinct types of symptoms, either diarrhoea without abdominal pain or an alternating pattern of diarrhoea and constipation with abdominal pain.

In addition to an altered bowel habit and abdominal pain, many other symptoms have been experienced by patients with irritable bowel syndrome (IBS). For example, nausea, flatulence, dysuria, dysmenorrhoea, fatigue, anxiety, depression, insomnia and irritability have been described by IBS patients (Eastwood *et al.*, 1987). Most of these symptoms are associated with stress, in fact psychological disorders have been recorded in over 90 per cent of patients with IBS (Hislop, 1971). In addition to stress many trigger factors have been thought to cause IBS, such as food allergy, gastro-intestinal infection, chronic alcohol abuse and bile salt malabsorption (Eastwood *et al.*, 1987). However, no specific organic disease has been attributed to the irregular bowel habits and abdominal pain characteristic of this disease (Manning *et al.*, 1978, Heaton, 1983).

The syndrome is more common in the 30–50 year age group and diagnosis normally requires the elimination of underlying organic disease (such as carcinoma, infection, Crohn's disease and diverticulitis) which could cause similar gastro-intestinal symptoms (Eastwood *et al.*, 1987). However, a positive diagnosis by the presenting symptoms rather than diagnosis by the exclusion of other diseases is becoming easier as experience is gained in identifying the characteristic gastro-intestinal abnormalities and emotional components of this illness (Harvey *et al.*, 1987). IBS is normally evaluated by the assessment of presenting symptoms, namely: abdominal distension, relief of pain with a bowel movement and frequent, looser stools at the onset of pain (Manning *et al.*, 1978). However, the emotional disturbances, although recognized, have yet to be formally assessed (Heaton, 1987).

Treatment is based on emotional reassurance and methods designed to modify intestinal functional. The fibre content of the diet is increased to relieve constipation and pain (Ritchie and Truelove, 1979). Painful diarrhoea is normally relieved with anticholinergic compounds such as dicyclomine or with an antispasmodic such as mebeverine (Crean *et al.*, 1984). The outcome of aggressive treatment based on adequate explanation of the illness, high-fibre diet, bulking agents such as ispaghula husk and antispasmodics is very good as about 85 per cent of patients can become symptom-free, of which almost 70 per cent remain symptom-free over five years later (Harvey *et al.*, 1987).

Assessment of IBS

In the assessment of IBS and the evaluation of pharmaceutical treatments, methods have focused on determining the extent of disruption of normal bowel habits and on the pain associated with the condition. The frequently occurring 'emotional symptoms' associated with IBS and subsequent effects on health and quality of life, although recognized, have not yet been fully identified or formally evaluated in most trials of therapy (Harvey *et al.*, 1987). There are no quality of life measures specifically designed to assess IBS. It was for this reason that the evaluation of health status in patients with IBS using the Nottingham

Health Profile was considered to be a valuable contribution both to the further validation of specific health status measures and to ascertaining whether such an evaluation provided an increased understanding of the effects of IBS on health and daily life.

This research was undertaken as part of a wide range of studies of health status assessment in various diseases including rheumatoid arthritis, osteoarthritis, angina, depression and cancer (Stevens *et al.*, 1986). The Nottingham Health Profile (NHP) was chosen as the most useful of all published health status indicators for the proposed studies because it covers a wide range of activities, is simple to administer and can be completed by the patient in less than ten minutes. The NHP consists of two parts. Part 1 consists of 38 questions describing health problems in terms of energy, sleep, pain, physical mobility, social isolation and emotions. Within each section of Part 1 the questions have been weighted according to perceived severity and can be combined to provide a profile of six scores to represent quality of life. Part 2 lists a number of areas which could be affected by health problems: job, household management, family life, sex life, social life, social life, holidays and hobbies. Previous investigations had shown it to be sensitive enough to evaluate health status in a wide range of situations including individual clinical interviews and population surveys (McEwen, 1983). Since it provides a comprehensive list of health problems with an emphasis on emotional aspects such as social isolation, sleep and emotions it was considered suitable to assess anxiety, depression and other emotional factors possibily associated with IBS. Validity and reliability were found to be very high during the development of the NHP (Beckett *et al.*, 1981). It was also considered applicable to clinical evaluations since it was inexpensive to administer and being self-completed by the patient substantially decreased the professional burden associated with data collection.

Objectives of the Research Project

The objectives of assessing health status in individuals suffering from IBS were threefold. The first was to determine the relationship between health status as measured by NHP scores, overall health as rated by patients and the usual clinical parameters used to assess IBS. The responses to the NHP would also enable the identification of areas in patients' lives and daily activities affected by IBS. Secondly, the study provided an opportunity to assess the ability of the NHP to differentiate between predictable variations in health status due to the varying degrees or severity of the clinical features of this syndrome. Finally, the most valuable part of the study was to assess the sensitivity of the NHP to clinical and overall health changes which result from consultation and the treatment of IBS.

Methods

One hundred and forty-six patients with IBS were recruited by thirty-seven general practitioners participating in multicentre study of the treatment of IBS using antispasmodics. Patients were interviewed and examined by the doctor and all other gastro-intestinal diseases had been excluded by radiological and other examinations. Thirty-five were male and one hundred and eleven were female—the median age was 36 years with a range of 18–53 years. In the week prior to commencing treatment, when the patients were interviewed and examined by the doctor, the following assessments were made: frequency of abdominal pain (number of pain episodes per 24 hours: none, less than five, six to ten, more than ten); severity of abdominal pain (none, mild, moderate, severe); type of bowel movement (loose with diarrhoea, hard and pellety, soft and formed). The patients also assessed their own health as very good, good, fair, poor or very poor and completed the NHP. They then received treatment with an antispasmodic and at the end of a four-week treatment period, all assessments were repeated. Participants also completed a second NHP and made a second assessment of their overall health. In addition, both the doctors and patients made a subjective assessment of the improvement in symptoms in terms of defecation pattern and abdominal pain (much worse, slightly worse, no change, slight improvement, great improvement).

Results

The frequency of positive responses to Parts I and II of the NHP are shown in Table 1. It can been seen that all activities of daily living measured by the NHP were affected by health problems arising from this disease but most individuals had health problems associated with emotions, energy and pain (as shown by Part I responses) and reported that their social life and home life were greatly affected by their current state of health. The majority of individuals (51 per cent) recorded their health as fair; abdominal pain severity was rated as mainly moderate or severe and the number of pain episodes varied in frequency from less than five episodes per day in 50 per cent of patients to more than ten per day in 10 per cent of patients (Table 2). The type of motion was described mainly as soft and formed by approximately 50 per cent of patients; an equivalent number reported hard, pellety stools or loose diarrhoeal stools (see Table 2 for pre-treatment scores for clinical parameters).

Table 1. Percentage of positive responses to the NHP in the pre-treatment (and post-treatment group shown in brackets)

Part I

Energy	%	(%)
I'm tired all the time	55	(21)
Everything is an effort	37	(20)
I soon run out of energy	58	(23)

Pain		
I have pain at night	66	(28)
I have unbearable pain	21	(7)
I find it painful to change position	23	(12)
I am in pain when I walk	35	(16)
I am in pain when I am standing	39	(17)
I am in constant pain	18	(7)
I am in pain when going up and down stairs	13	(7)
I am in pain when sitting	40	(19)

Emotions		
Things are getting me down	68	(31)
I have forgotten what it is like to enjoy myself	38	(14)
I am feeling on edge	66	(42)
The days seem to drag	31	(18)
I lose my temper easily	62	(36)
I feel as if I am losing control	24	(8)
Worry is keeping me awake	31	(22)
I feel that life is not worth living	10	(4)
I wake up feeling depressed	36	(19)

Social isolation		
I feel lonely	19	(14)
I am finding it hard to make contact with people	11	(9)
I feel there is nobody I am close to	15	(9)
I feel I am a burden to people	14	(6)
I am finding it hard to get on with people	19	(8)

Sleep		
I take tablets to help me sleep	16	(14)
I am waking in the early hours of the morning	54	(30)
I am awake most of the night	19	(11)
It takes me a long time to get to sleep	45	(32)
I sleep badly at night	43	(29)

Physical mobility		
I can only walk around indoors	6	(1)
I find it hard to bend	31	(15)
I am unable to walk at all	0	(0)
I find steps and stairs difficult	6	(6)
I find it hard to reach for things	14	(9)
I find it hard to dress	3	(3)
I find it hard to stand for long	43	(27)
I need help to walk outside	1	(1)

Part II

	Job	Housework	Social life	Home life	Sex life	Interests	Holidays
%(%)	37(24)	43(23)	53(21)	49(23)	38(20)	38(18)	34(19)

Table 2. Percentage scores of clinical parameters: Patient-rated pre-treatment and post-treatment

Patient-rated overall health	Pre-treatment	Post-treatment
Very good	7	16
Good	29	51
Fair	51	26
Poor	13	5
Very poor	0	2

Severity of abdominal pain	Pre-treatment	Post-treatment
None	6	42
Mild	27	44
Moderate	52	12
Severe	15	2

Number of pain episodes per day	Pre-treatment	Post-treatment
None	5	35
Less than five	50	57
Six to ten	35	6
More than ten	10	1

Type of motion	Pre-treatment	Post-treatment
Hard and pellety	30	12
Loose with diarrhoea	23	5
Soft and formed	47	83

Relationship between Health Status and Clinical Measures

Various statistical analyses were performed in order to determine the relationship between clinical and health scores in the pre-treatment group of individuals. The data from this study were skewed rather than normally distributed with frequently recorded scores at the lower and upper limits, so non-parametric statistical tests were used as the criteria required for parametic tests were not met (Siegel, 1959). There were no age and sex differences in health status scores for this population (Spearman's rank correlation coefficients in all comparisons were <0.3).

Clinical and NHP scores were compared for the four health categories: very good, good, fair, poor. There was a close relationship between the participants' perception of their overall health and NHP Part 1 scores for pain, emotion, energy and physical mobility ($P < 0.05$, using Kruskall–Wallis one-way analysis of variance), but not for social isolation or sleep ($P > 0.05$). However, clinical scores for abdominal pain frequency and severity did not significantly relate to overall health status ($P > 0/1$).

NHP scores were compared for each measured clinical parameter score. Patient-related abdominal pain severity and frequency showed a positive relationship (P <0.01, Kruskall–Wallis one-way ANOVA) whereas there was no significant difference in NHP or overall health scores for the four categories of patient-rated or physician-rated abdominal pain severity or to the severity of the routinely measured clinical parameters.

The Effects of Treatment

One of the primary objectives of this study was to determine the sensitivity of the NHP to clinical change which results from the treatment of IBS. The post-treatment scores shown in Table 3 were compared with the pre-treatment values by means of non-parametric statistical tests.

The post-treatment scores for the clinical parameters (also shown in Table 2) indicate that this group of patients generally had no pain or mild abdominal pain and more than half experienced less than five episodes of pain per day following treatment. The consistency of stools had also improved to 'soft and

Table 3. Improvement in abdominal pain (and defecation pattern) as judged by patient and physician

	Much worse	Slightly worse	No change	Slight improvement	Great improvement
Patient-related abdominal pain					
Percentage	1	3	9	40	47
Physician-rated abdominal pain					
Percentage	0	1	10	36	52
Patient-rated defecation pattern					
Percentage	0	2	18	34	46
Physician-rated defecation pattern					
Percentage	0	3	14	37	46

formed' for over 80 per cent of the population. Overall health scores at this assessment were 'good' for more than 50 per cent of the population. Results in Table 1 show that the percentage of affirmative responses to both parts of NHP had generally decreased, indicating an improvement in patients' perception of health. Although the problems still existed for this patient population, they appeared to be less common after treatment.

The pre-treatment and post-treatment scores for clinical parameters, overall health and the NHP were compared by means of Wilcoxon's matched pairs signed ranks test. Results are shown in Figure 1 (abdominal pain severity and frequency; Figure 2 (patient-rated overall health); Figure 3 (NHP Part I scores) and Figure 4 (NHP Part II scores). These figures illustrate that post-treatment scores for all patient were significantly lower than those for the pre-treatment assessment (Wilcoxon's matched pairs signed rank test $P < 0.01$). This indicates a general improvement in all clinical symptoms and in general well-being determined from overall health scores and both parts of the NHP.

In Part I of the NHP, scores for emotions and pain were the most sensitive to clinical improvement in IBS, while scores for social isolation, sleep and physical mobility were less sensitive to these identified clinical changes. Patients and doctors participating in this study made judgements on changes in abdominal pain and defecation pattern at the post-treatment assessment shown in Table 3. Both patient- and doctor-rated abdominal pain and defecation pattern were considered to have slightly or greatly improved for more than 80 per cent of the population.

Discussion

This study has contributed further experience in the clinical use of the Nottingham Health Profile. This health status profile was able to identify health-related problems particularly associated with energy, emotional reactions and pain in this population. These health problems decreased most significantly as a result of treatment whereas there were smaller changes in the health problems of physical mobility, sleep and social isolation which were considered to be less severe in this population. From the study it is not possible to differentiate the improvement that occurred as a result of the care in clinical consultation from that produced by treatment with antispasmodics. However, the addition of the NHP has provided information about emotional 'distress' in this population, which is not routinely assessed as part of the clinical examination.

While health status indicators have been used for many aspects of health care evaluation, it is only recently that they have found a place in the assessment of pharmaceutical treatment. Wider acceptance of health status indicators in routine clinical evaluation depends upon further research and the publication of such studies to bring them to the attention of the clinicians and others conduct-

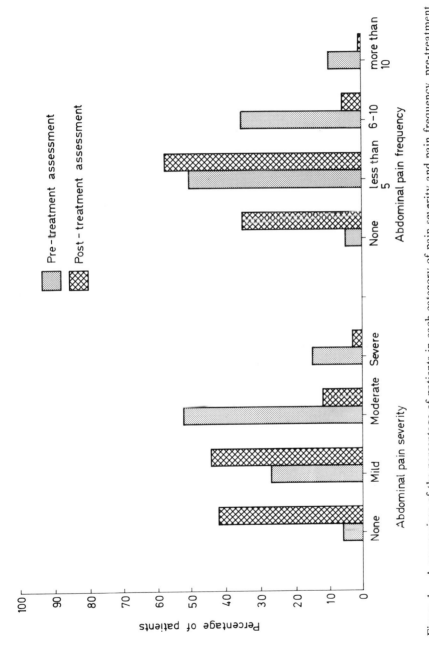

Figure 1. A comparison of the percentage of patients in each category of pain severity and pain frequency, pre-treatment and post-treatment

220

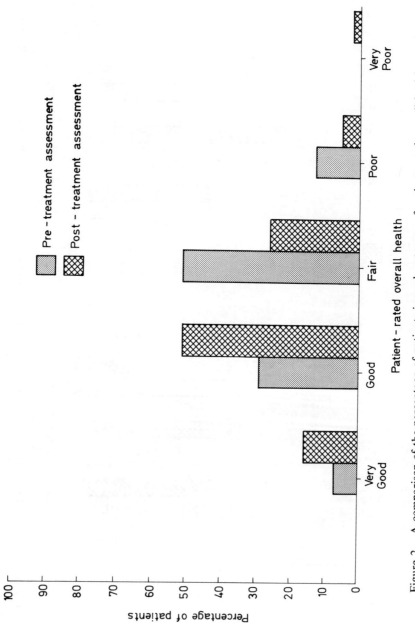

Figure 2. A comparison of the percentage of patients in each category of patient-rated overall health, pre-treatment and post-treatment

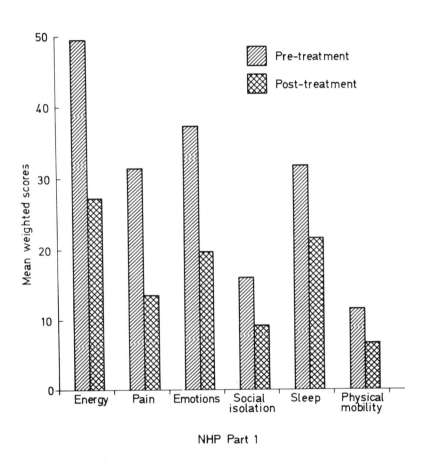

Figure 3. A comparison of pre-treatment and post-treatment scores for NHP Part I

ing such investigations. Only then will the addition of health status assessment become established as a valuable adjunct to clinical evaluation. The use of the NHP and other quality of life measures will allow more consideration to be given by the doctor to those aspects of health perceived to be important by the patients. Above all, the assessment of health status in diseases such as IBS could make a valuable contribution to decisions with regard to treatment.

222

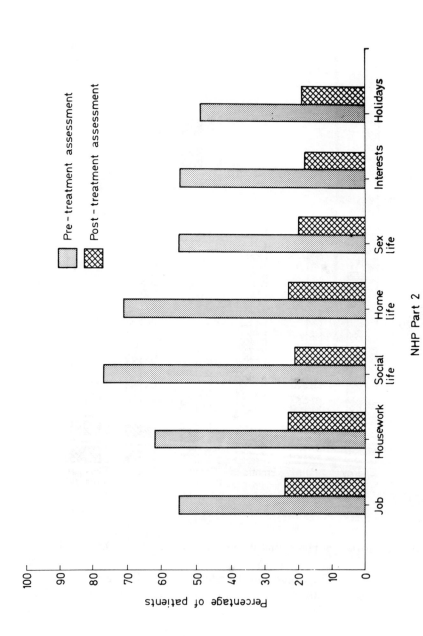

Figure 4. A comparison of the percentage of patients who gave affirmative responses to part 2 of the NHP, pre-treatment and post-treatment

Acknowledgements

The authors would like to acknowledge the important contribution of Dr D. Williams (Reckitt and Colman) who stimulated our interest in this disease, Dr P. Weedle (Welsh School of Pharmacy, UWIST) for help with computing statistical analyses and Dr J. M. McEwen (King's College Hospital Medical School) for allowing us to use the Nottingham Health Profile in this study.

References

Backett, E. M. *et al.* (1981). Health and Quality of Life—*end of grant report No HR 6157/1*, London: Social Science Research Council.

Crean, G. P. *et al.* (1984). Diseases of the alimentary tracts and pancreas. In *Davidson's Principles and Practice of Medicine*, ed. MacLeod, J., London: Churchill Livingstone.

Eastwood, M. A. *et al.* (1987). The irritable bowel syndrome: a disease or a response? Discussion paper. *Journal of the Royal Society of Medicine*, **80**, 219–21.

Harvey, R. F. *et al.* (1987). Prognosis of the irritable bowel syndrome, a five year prospective study. *Lancet*, **25**, 963–5.

Heaton, K. W. (1983). Irritable bowel syndrome: still in search of its identity. *British Medical Journal*, **287**, 852–3.

Hislop, I. G. (1971). Psychological significance of the irritable colon syndrome. *Gut*, **12**, 452–5.

Manning, A. P. *et al.* (1978). Towards a positive diagnosis of irritable bowel syndrome. *British Medical Journal*, 2 September, 653–4.

McEwen, J. (1983). The Nottingham Health Profile. In *Measuring the Social Benefits of Medicines*, ed. Teeling-Smith, G., London: OHE.

Ritchie, J. A. and Truelove, S. C. (1979). Treatment of irritable bowel syndrome with lorazepam, hyoscine butylbromide and ispaghula husk. *British Medical Journal*, **1**, 376–8.

Siegel, S. (1959). *Non-parametric Statistics for the Behavioural Sciences*, Tokyo: McGraw-Hill.

Stevens, J. C. *et al.* (1986). Is quality of life important and measurable during clinical evaluation? *British Journal of Clinical Pharmacology*, **22**(2), 245.

Measuring Health: A Practical Approach
Edited by G. Teeling Smith
© 1988 John Wiley & Sons Ltd

11

Applications in Management

Alan Williams
Department of Economics, University of York

Introduction

The key difference between the decisions of clinicians and the decisions of managers is that the former concern choice of treatment (here and now) for a particular individual, while the latter concern choice of treatment facilities for a whole community of (current and future) patients. In both cases issues of cost, life expectancy and quality of life will be relevant (Williams, 1984) but they will present themselves in a different context, and may need to be treated in a different way. For instance, in a particular clinical context, more detailed knowledge of the effects of treatments on particular aspects of quality of life may be needed than for a managerial decision on broad priorities, but the *range* of quality of life characteristics that is relevant may be broader in the management context than in the clinical context, since the different conditions/treatments that are being compared (e.g. dental care vs hernia repair) may affect rather different aspects of people's lives. In general, therefore, the application of quality of life measurement in a management context will inevitably be more 'broad brush' than in a clinical context. This means that for resource management purposes it will be necessary to find a way of *describing* quality of life which concentrates on features of illness which are commonly experienced with a wide variety of treatments and conditions, yet which make sense equally well in each of these contexts.

Unfortunately, management decision-making is also much more demanding in its information requirements with respect to valuation. Quality of life measurement involves both the description and the relative valuation of different health states. At a clinical level it could be argued that the valuation issue is easily solved (in principle, at any rate) by asking the patient (with respect to different treatment options) which is the preferred outcome profile (in terms of life expectancy and quality of life). But for management purposes this is not enough. We also need to know *how much* better one treatment is than another, *and* how benefits to one person are to be weighed against that same benefit to another person. (This latter issue has in fact also to be faced by every clinician, in his role as practice manager, though many clinicians seem unaware that they are doing this, and often even vehemently deny doing it.)

The reason for these additional requirements is that the problem management faces is that no health care system has enough resources to be able to provide *all* the facilities that might *possibly* improve *someone's* life expectancy or quality of life. Because of this inescapable resource constraint, some beneficial procedures cannot be undertaken, so criteria need to be established to determine which shall have priority, and the natural reaction is to concentrate on those that do the *most* good. Hence the necessity of measuring the *relative value* of the benefits to be gained by providing different facilities, so that these benefits can be compared with the costs of generating them. This rules out quality of life measures which stop at the stage of generating 'profiles' (e.g. the Nottingham Health Profile).

Since the focus of interest in this book is on benefit measurement rather than on cost measurement, no further consideration will be given to the resource measurement side of the manager's problem, important though it is. It will simply be assumed that there exists an estimated cost per patient treated, based on precisely the same comparison as is being made on the benefit side. This requires a careful specification of what precisely is being compared. For instance, is it one treatment vs another treatment, or treatment vs no treatment? And what is the time span of the comparison? Is it simply the immediate episode of illness or treatment, or does it cover all consequential commitments, for example follow-up clinics, risks of readmission, and continuing aftercare (possibly for the rest of a patient's life)? Clearly it will be misleading to compute benefits over the rest of a patient's life but costs only for the immediate episode of treatment (or vice-versa).

Finally, it is assumed here that what is required is guidance on the best methods to use from amongst those that are already available, with minimal additional work. Nevertheless, no one should embark on the task of measuring quality of life believing that it is a simple mechanical process which will churn out data in a routine or comprehensive manner. It is best tackled at present where well-structured choices have to be made and where there is time to put in some skilled effort and thought.

The Practical Task

Against that background, the practical task of estimating the relative value of different treatments can be broken down into several stages, each of which will be tackled in turn. These are:

1. Choosing a suitable framework for describing quality of life.
2. Gathering data that can be fitted into this framework.
3. (Generating and) using a set of valuations to rate these different quality of life states relatively to each other.
4. Incorporating an explicit trade-off between quality of life and life expectancy
5. Deciding on what basis gains to one person are to be compared with identical gains to another person.

Choosing a Descriptive Framework

The criteria to be applied here are:

i. is the framework applicable to a suitably wide range of treatments or conditions?
ii. does it have a suitably derived set of relative valuations which can be used with it? (see below for further consideration of this point);
iii. has it already been used as a basis for a great deal of information collection relevant to the choices under consideration?
iv. how easy will it be to supplement such data by fitting into the framework data collected for other purposes?
v. can new data easily be collected specifically to fill gaps in the existing data?

Points iii, iv and v will be considered in more detail in the next section.

At present there are very few well worked out global indexes of health. The leading contenders for use at a managerial level are the Sickness Impact Profile, the Quality of Well-Being Scale, the McMaster Health Index Questionnaire and the Rosser Index, all of which are reviewed by Kind (Chapter 3) in this volume. Amongst these, the only one of which I have direct experience is that due to Rosser. It has the advantage of being the simplest to understand and use (and, for British applications, the additional advantage that its valuations were derived from British respondents, a point to be reviewed later). I shall therefore concentrate exclusively on Rosser's classification (see Table 1), though similar considerations would apply if one of the others were chosen as the preferred starting point.

Table 1. Rosser's classification of states of ill-health

Disability		Distress	
I.	No disability	A.	Distress
II.	Slight social disability	B.	Mild
III.	Severe social disability and/or slight impairment of performance at work.	C.	Moderate
	Able to do all housework except very heavy tasks	D.	Severe
IV.	Choice of work or performance at work very severely limited.		
	Housewives and old people able to do light housework only but able to go out shopping		
V.	Unable to undertake any paid employment.		
	Unable to continue any education.		
	Old people confined to home except for escorted outings and short walks and unable to do shopping.		
	Housewives able only to perform a few simple tasks		
VI.	Confined to chair or to wheelchair or able to move around in the house only with support from an assistant		
VII.	Confined to bed		
VIII.	Unconscious		

Gathering Descriptive Data

There are essentially four ways of gathering data for use in the Rosser classification of illness states. The first is to use data that someone else has already collected within that classification system. At present such data are sparse (see Williams, 1987a) and unlikely to cover the precise range of options that is being considered in some specific context. It is, therefore, almost inevitably that one or more of the other three methods will have to be used, namely, reclassification of data collected according to some other classification system; professional judgement as to the likely distribution of outcomes across the Rosser states; or *ad hoc* surveys of patients (e.g. by questionnaire) to elicit their appropriate place in the Rosser classification.

Reclassification of other people's data requires, first of all, that the literature be searched for studies reporting on quality of life outcomes for the relevant conditions and treatments. The actual dimensions of quality of life measured in each study then need to be examined closely to see how exactly they correspond to Rosser's categories, and some rules need to be established for determining what is to be regarded as equivalent to what. This is bound to be a matter of judgement. Examples of such 'translations' are given in Gudex (1986). It is a process in which some information is bound to be lost, because *either* the source will have more detail than Rosser's classification, and some of the source data will be more sketchy than Rosser's classification, and some of Rosser's categories will need to be compressed to accommodate this fact.

As an example, consider the following source data (Bonney *et al.*, 1978). In this study patients' physical activity was graded according to the US National Kidney Foundation Classification, and the corresponding Rosser disability grades appear to be as indicated:

National Kidney Foundation Classification		Corresponding Rosser Disability Grade
Class	Description	
1	Capable of performing all usual types of physical activity	I–II
2	Unable to perform the most strenuous of usual physical activities, e.g. sports, lawn mowing	III
3	Unable to perform usual daily activities on more than a part-time basis, e.g. housework, employment	IV
4	Severe limitation of usual physical activity May be confined to bed	V–VIII

The patients also completed questionnaires of the Kupfer–Detre System, which evaluates current psychological states and elicits the presence or absence of specific physical symptoms. It generates a depression score in which a rating ≥ 10 is said to represent severe depression. Thus the following correspondence may be used as a working hypothesis:

KDS Depression Score	Rosser Distress Category
<8	A/B
≥ 8 but ≤ 10	C
>10	D

Unfortunately this published study did not report the distribution of patients across both dimensions in a single table, but only for each dimension separately, so further assumptions are then required, for example that the more disabled patients tend to be the more depressed. Sometimes further distributions can be obtained by writing to the authors. Otherwise the only practicable way forward is to test how sensitive the overall outcome is to working with different plausible assumptions.

If it is impossible to find relevant descriptive data on quality of life in the published literature (and it is surprisingly scarce) the next possibility to consider is getting some expert opinions canvassed systematically. Clearly this is not as good as relying on the results of large well-designed randomized controlled trials, but there are not many of those about, and if the treatment is relatively new, and the required follow-up time is quite long, there may be no alternative but to rely on 'informed opinions' or 'expert judgement', in this and in other aspects of treatment effectiveness. The important thing is to elicit such judgements from people whom you have good reason to suppose are the more knowledgeable, and who are *either* unbiased as individuals or, if this is impossible, whose known biases offset each other if you are able to canvass the views of more than one person (which is definitely to be recommended).

The Rosser classification scheme can be used to elicit likely prognoses by using the format set out in Table 2, in which the respondent (say a clinician or medical researcher specializing in the field) is asked to provide two prognoses for each specified condition and patient type. The one prognosis would be for one treatment, and the other for the alternative (which may be no treatment). There may of course be more than two treatment options, and a variety of patient types, and various different manifestations of the condition (e.g. by stage of development, or site, etc.). The respondent is asked to supply data on how the patient's quality of life is expected to be affected over succeeding periods (e.g. weeks, months or years, according to which time horizon is appropriate in the specific circumstances) by completing the grid. An example is shown on Tables 3a and 3b which are the views of a cardiac surgeon concerning the relative outcomes to be expected from CABG or medical management for moderate angina.

Obviously, if this process yields widely different views from different respondents, the possibility opens up for an intriguing dialogue between the parties concerned (see Williams, 1987b). For immediate policy-making purposes, however, the objective of such a dialogue should be *either* to seek some kind of expert consensus, *or* to determine the range of alternative views it might be prudent to include in a sensitivity analysis.

The final possibility, if the foregoing methods of gathering descriptive data have failed, or have left gaps which need to be filled, is to gather such data directly oneself. Unless research capacity is available, the best one can hope for may be one can get access, at a point in time, to a sizeable number of patients who will have been treated in various ways at varying times in the past. Such retrospective (cross-sectional) data will then have to be taken as an approximation to the (longitudinal) quality of life profile for the relevant

Table 2. Estimating outcomes by clinical judgement

Principal diagnosis . . . .

Other significant concurrent conditions . . . .

. . . .

. . . .

Severity indicators . . . .

. . . .

Age . . . . Sex . . . .

Treatment A   *Treatment B*

. . . .

* Perioperative mortality rate (%) ......   * Perioperative mortality rate (%) ......

Proportion of patients who do not   Proportion of patients who do not
respond to treatment (%)   ......   respond to treatment (%)   ......

Increase in life expectancy of   Increase in life expectancy of
patients who do respond to   patients who do respond to
treatment (years)   ......   treatment (years)   ......

Notes: Place '0' on each grid to represent the typical state of a patient at the time of referral (thus it should be identically placed on both grids).

Thereafter denote by 1, 2, 3, ... etc. the state in which you would expect a successfully treated patient to be at each successive annual interval thereafter, ceasing with the year corresponding to average life expectancy.

* To be completed if a treatment involves surgery.

Table 3. One clinician's estimates of outcome in the treatment of angina pectoria

CONDITION .MODERATE. . . . ANGINA WITH ..2... VESSEL DISEASE

(Male, aged 55 years) .LESION. PROXIMAL. . . . .

A. MEDICAL MANAGEMENT

Av. life expectancy 10 YEARS

B. CABG

Perioperative mortality ..1... %

Average life expectancy .15... years
(excluding perioperative mortality)

Cases where no symptomatic relief ..5... %

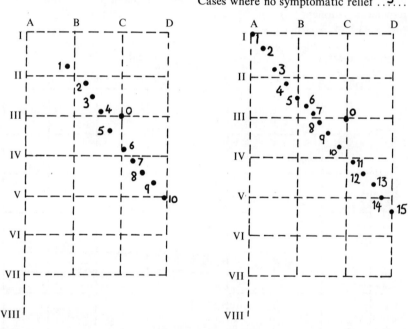

Notes: Place '0' on each grid to represent the typical state of a patient at the time of referral (thus it should be identically placed on both grids).

Thereafter denote by 1, 2, 3, ... etc. the state in which you would expect a successfully treated patient to be at each successive annual interval thereafter, ceasing with the year corresponding to average life expectancy.

condition, treatment, and patient type. Using the Rosser classification, a quite simple, self-assessed questionnaire (as in Annexe A) can be used to do this, using a set of rules (as in Annexe B) to classify the responses into the Rosser matrix. It should be remembered, however, that this method will not pick up the non-survivors, whose respective lengths of life will need to have been recorded separately. It may also miss those who are too seriously ill to be able to respond, so these biases may need to be adjusted for.

Relative Valuations

Assuming that by one means or another it has been possible to generate a table of outcomes, described in Rosser terms, for each treatment option, the next stage is to attach to each an index of relative value. The convention used in this valuation index is that being healthy is rated at 1, and being dead at 0, so that such a valuation index must permit some living states to be rated as being as bad as (or possibly worse than) being dead, that is, zero, or even negative, ratings are possible.

Rosser's classification scheme has the great advantage that it had just such a valuation matrix to go with it, and this is set out in Table 4. It does have its limitations, however, amongst which are that it was derived from only 70 subjects, who were not a representative sample of the population. Details of the respondents, and some analysis of the valuations of different subgroups, are to be found in Rosser and Kind (1978), and Kind *et al.* (1982). Two such subgroups' valuations are shown in Tables 5a and 5b. If the data in Tables 3a and 3b were valued according to the views of Rossers' 70 respondents, then they could be represented as shown in Figure 1. This sort of comparison was pursued further in Williams (1985).

The prudent pragmatic way forward here may well be to test the sensitivity of the outcomes to the use of each of these valuation matrices, for it may well be that the specific options under consideration are always rated much the same, relatively to each other, whichever set of valuations is used (especially when the relative cost data are also brought into the picture).

But if the choice does seem to depend critically upon the particular choice of valuation matrix from amongst Rossers' subgroups, or if it is desired to replace it with one reflecting the views of other people, then consideration should be given to possible ways of eliciting such values from whoever are regarded as the appropriate respondents.

This matter of who is the appropriate respondents is, of course, at bottom a political decision (as to whose valued shall count) so it is not for me to say who they should be. But there are points to bear in mind about each of the obvious caididates. Patients themselves are usually the first group who spring to mind, but if you are comparing competing claims for facilities for, say, renal dialysis, hip replacements, coronary artery bypass grafting, and AIDS, *which* patients'

Table 4. Rosser's valuation matrix (all 70 respondents)

Disability rating	Distress rating			
	A	B	C	D
I	1.000	0.995	0.990	0.967
II	0.990	0.986	0.973	0.932
III	0.980	0.972	0.956	0.912
IV	0.964	0.956	0.942	0.870
V	0.946	0.935	0.900	0.700
VI	0.875	0.845	0.680	0.000
VII	0.677	0.564	0.000	−1.486
VIII	−1.028			

Table 5. Rosser's valuation matrix (doctors and medical patients)

A. Doctors ($N = 10$)

Disability \ Distress	1	2	3	4
1	1.000	0.992	0.946	0.793
2	0.981	0.973	0.865	0.766
3	0.946	0.913	0.848	0.668
4	0.923	0.888	0.760	0.187
5	0.873	0.865	0.692	−0.394
6	0.800	0.773	0.298	−0.803
7	0.505	0.452	0.000	−2.288
8	−1.077			

B. Medical patients ($N = 10$)

Disability \ Distress	1	2	3	4
1	1.000	0.992	0.986	0.977
2	0.987	0.982	0.968	0.936
3	0.980	0.966	0.958	0.915
4	0.954	0.951	0.937	0.893
5	0.924	0.910	0.903	0.840
6	0.863	0.848	0.760	0.440
7	0.640	0.371	0.000	−1.480
8	−0.422			

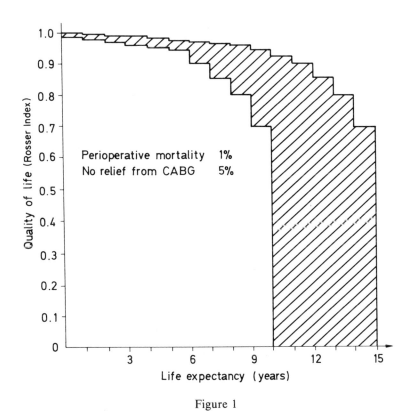

Figure 1

views do you canvass, and what weight do you give to each, and WHY? Also, each patient will have an incentive to respond in whatever way is believed likely to attract resources in his or her direction (though in fact it is quite difficult to know just what 'false signals' are optimal in this situation). It may be further objected that patients will not have experienced most of the states (or even observed others in them very frequently) so a better informed set of values might be elicited from doctors or nurses. But they too have a special interest, and there is plenty of evidence suggesting generally that doctors' beliefs about what patients care about often differ significantly from what patients actually care about. But then there is another consideration to be borne in mind in a managerial context, namely that it is the resources of the taxpayers (i.e. of the citizenry at large) that are at stake here, so maybe it should be their views that count. They are more likely to be able to take a deliberative view, and less likely to be emotionally involved in a specific situation, than either the patients or the health care professionals. But they may also suffer from lack of experience, so maybe it would be better to rely on their representatives, especially those specifically charged with determining priorities in health care, that is members of health authorities or others with political accountability to the citizenry at large. It is not a straightforward matter deciding whose values to elicit.

Eliciting these values is essentially a research task if it is to be done rigorously, but it would be possible to get a rough idea whether any selected group of respondents approximated the views of the Rosser respondents (or any subset thereof) in the following manner. Prepare 29 cards on each of which is described one of the Rosser illness states (i.e. one for each possible combination of disability and distress, except that the state 'unconscious' is not differentiated with respect to distress). Ask respondents to put these in order from best to worst. Then ask whether, if they faced the prospect of being in each such state for the rest of their lives, they would regard any of the states as being just about as bad as being dead. If any states are so nominated, they are rated at 0 for that respondent. Then respondents generally are told to take the state 'no disability and no distress' as worth 1, and the state dead as worth zero, and to rate all the other states accordingly, according to how bad they seem relatively to these fixed points. Obviously a negative weight will be given to any states that were ranked worse than a state which was nominated as being as bad as being dead. This crude experiment could either be done on an individual basis and the responses collected by the investigator, or if conducted with the members of (say) a health authority, they could be encouraged to talk through their differences (if any) and come to a common view as to what valuation matrix should be used as constituting the policy of the authority.

They may, in the end, of course, decide to go back to the values of Rosser's 70 respondents!

Quality of Life vs Quantity of Life

The essence of a global index which works with dead = 0 and healthy = 1 is that it involves systematic comparison of the value of changes in life expectancy compared with changes in quality of life.

Indeed that is why such indices have tended to develop into quality adjustment factors for use with life expectancy to generate the composite measure known generically as the quality-adjusted life-year or QALY.

Such a trade-off is already buried away in the Rosser valuation matrix (Table 4 above). Consider the state VIIA, which is rated at 0.677 (approximately two-thirds). This could be interpreted as meaning that the individual in question is indifferent between the prospect of three years in that state or two years of good health (State IA, rated at 1). Put another way, this individual would be prepared to sacrifice up to one year's life expectancy in every three to improve his or her quality of life from VIIA to IA. Other possible moves in the Rosser matrix could be similarly interpreted.

In fact the QALY calculation is somewhat more complex than simply applying this valuation matrix because the distribution of outcomes is not certain, but probabilistic, so that in Figure 1, for instance, the hatched gain is expected to be enjoyed by only 95 per cent of treated patients (5 per cent no gain), while an unfortunate 1 per cent lose (through perioperative mortality) the benefits they would have enjoyed had they stuck with medical management (as represented by the clear area below the lower boundary of the hatched area). A further complication is that benefits in the future (like costs in the future) need to be discounted at some appropriate rate (say 5 per cent) to reflect the fact that people generally prefer benefits sooner rather than later (and costs later rather than sooner).

Interpersonal Comparisons

As with all measures of effectiveness, the relevant data are for groups rather than for an individual, and hence involve some (often implicit) weighting of benefits between people. For instance, the common use of the two-year survival rate as the criterion for choosing between treatment implies (i) that to survive less than 2 years is of no value to anybody, (ii) to survive beyond two years is of no additional benefit to anybody, (iiii) providing you survive two years it does not matter with what quality of life you survive, and (iv) survival to two years is of equal value to everybody.

A measure such as the Rosser QALY is more sensitive than this, in that it counts *all* additional life expectancy, does not impose any arbitrary cut-off-point, and it adjusts for differential quality of life expectancy. But in its straightforward use it assumes that being dead is equally bad for everybody (since dead = 0 is a convention to which everyone's valuations conform) and being healthy is equally good for everybody (since healthy = 1 is also a convention common to everybody's valuations). The implications of this are that one year of healthy life expectancy is regarded as of equal value to everybody. So (subject to the complication mentioned earlier about discounting to take account of remoteness) one extra healthy year for each of ten people is regarded as of equal value to an extra 10 healthy years for one person. This is quite a strong (specific) egalitarian position, which is *either* acceptable as a suitable expression of policy *or* it is not. If it is acceptable, then QALYs can simply be added together no matter who gets them.

But if it is *not* acceptable a more complicated process would have to take place at this point. First of all, a more acceptable ethical position would have to be formulated (e.g. that QALYs for old people should count for more than if they were for young people, or for men vs women, or for rich vs poor, or for 'productive' vs 'unproductive', or whatever is thought to be more ethical than all QALYs being of equal value). Then the impact of different treatments upon each different subset would have to be identified. Then it would have to be decided what the differential weight should be (e.g. 1.1 for an old folk's QALY, but 0.9 for a young person, or vice-versa). These distinctions can be as complicated as is necessary and feasible, but they will need to be made explicit and justified to the relevant policy-makers.

Concluding Observations

The practical task of gathering, processing and deploying data on differential quality of life outcomes in health care is no easy task, and it requires careful focusing on clearly formulated decisions. Thus rather than simply asking 'what is the quality of life of patients after treatment X?', one has to specify 'compared with what?'. Moreover, it is also important to know what are the characteristics of the patients who will be treated by treatment X (instead of the alternative treatment) for it may well be that they will differ from the patients who are currently being so treated (the history of most therapies is that they start off being used only on the most favourable cases, but as capacity expands, less and less promising cases are taken on board, so that the marginal benefits of extending capacity are lower than the average benefits achieved with existing cases).

In the present state of knowledge, I would not recommend attempting blanket coverage of a wide range of conditions and treatments, but concentrating on two kinds of management decision as the focus for particular attention. The first of these is when a bid is being made for special funding of some expensive therapy (which may well be technology-led) where, because of the size of the funds involved, a rather formal and deliberative decision process is involved. In such a case, the bidders should be required to produce evidence of expected benefit to patients, in terms of survival and/or quality of life, by one or other of the methods outlined here.

The other kind of management decision in which immediate progress might be easier than elsewhere, is in the annual cycle of allocation of funds to different specialties. Here it would be a matter of taking the main blocks of work within each speciality, and asking the clinicians to rate each of them roughly by the amount of benefit generated per unit of resource used (e.g. by bed day, or by operating theatre time, or by consultant time, or by generalized cost, whichever is the key resource constraint on which resource allocation decisions are focused). Then, with this rank ordering to hand for each specialty, ask what *extra* work, not being undertaken at present, they would regard as the most beneficial (in the same terms as above). Then, for each specialty, generate some more specific data, of the QALY type, on the *least* beneficial things they are doing at present, and the *most* beneficial things they are *not doing* at present. If *within* a specialty the latter is better than the former, get them to change their priorities. But *across* specialities, give precedence to those where the benefits at the margin are greatest per unit of resource.

If one wants to be even more adventurous, it might also be useful to apply these ideas to the much misunderstood issue of waiting lists. Popular folklore treats the size of waiting lists as evidence of unmet need and therefore as a source of guidance as to where the NHS patients need additional resources. Slightly more sophisticated folklore deals in waiting *times* rather than the *size* of lists, but otherwise is indistinguishable from the popular folklore. The cognoscenti are wary of all waiting list data because

i. they are not systematically related to how active a particular consultant is;
ii. the rate at which patients get onto lists is largely in the hands of the consultant with the list;
iii. some patients are put on a list as a substitute for telling them to wait and see if the condition sorts itself out without further treatment, and for this purpose a longish wait may be optimal;
iv. up to a point, it is better for patients (and everyone else) for them to be on a list than not on a list;
v. doctors interested in private practice find long NHS waiting times profitable.

Is there then *anything* useful for priority setting in the NHS that can be extracted from waiting lists? The answer is 'Yes' if the following statements seem a reasonable summary of the clinical situation:

1. The urgency associated with any elective treatment is a matter of degree in which patients fall along a *continuum*.
2. Clinicians are good at judging where on this continuum anyone is at any point in time and moderately good at judging how stable that position is (i.e. whether the proposed treatment of a patient's condition is getting more or less urgent, or staying roughly constant).
3. There may be an 'optimum' time for treatment, before which it is 'too soon' and after which it is 'too late'.
4. Clinicians wish to use their treatment capacity to the full, and to concentrate it on those patients who will benefit most from it.

In such circumstances the patients on a waiting list at any one time should be rated according to their capacity to benefit from treatment per unit of the constrained treatment resource, as indicated by the expected improvement (and as measured by QALYs). Those expected to get the greatest improvements should be given priority. A particular patient's capacity to benefit may change through time, and should, therefore, be reviewed as necessary.

If every clinician is pursuing this policy, then additional resources should be given to those clinicians whose *marginal* patients (i.e. those treated clients who benefit *least* from treatment) are gaining more from treatment than anyone else. That means that if the marginal patients of specialty X are getting

3 QALYS from treatment (and they have more such patients on their waiting lists) then that specialty would get priority over specialty Y, if the latter's marginal patients (and those at the head of the waiting list) would only get 1 QALY from treatment. Thus the key element about the waiting list is the nature of the patients on it. A specialty with a *small* list of people waiting a *short* time for a *very beneficial* treatment should have priority over one with a *long* list of patients who have been on it for *ages* but who will *benefit very little* from the treatment even when they get it.

With this approach to waiting lists clinicians will no longer have an incentive to expand their lists unrealistically in the hope of obtaining more resources, but instead will concentrate on keeping waiting times convenient for patients (i.e. just long enough to enable them to get themselves sorted out and minimize the disruptions to their lives caused by their treatment). And as resources are redirected to the more beneficial procedures, the use of waiting lists as a surreptitious 'wait and see' policy should cease, and there should be less incentive for patients to have recourse to the private sector for any of the more beneficial treatments that the NHS provides.

There is thus plenty of scope for imaginative, skilful, and persistent managers (from clinical practice level to national policy level) to employ quality of life measurement to tackle many of the resource allocation problems in running health care systems that have hitherto proved quite intractable.

References

Bonney, S. *et al*. (1978). Treatment of end-stage renal failure in a defined geographical area. *Arch. Intern. Med.*, **138**, 1510–3.

Gudex, C. (1986). QALYs and their use by the Health Service. University of York, Centre for Health Economics, Discussion Paper 20.

Kind, P., Rosser, R. and Williams, A. (1982). Valuation of quality of life: some psychometric evidence. In *The Value of Life and Safety* (ed. Jones-Lee, M. WE., Amsterdam: North-Holland.

Rosser, R. and Kind, P. (1978). A scale of valuations of states of illness: if there a social consensus?. *Inst. J. of Epidemiology* **6–7**, 347–58.

Williams, A. (1984). Medical ethics. In *Nuffield/York Portfolios*, ed. Culyer, A. J., Nuffield Provincial Hospitals Trust.

Williams, A. (1985). The economics of coronary artery bypass grafting. *Brit. Med. J.*, **291**, 325–9.

Williams, A. (1987a). The importance of 'Quality of Life' in policy decisions. In *Quality of Life: Assesment and Application*, ed. Walker, S. R., MTP Press.

Williams, A. (1987b). The cost effectiveness approach to the treatment of angina. In *The Management of Angina Pectoris*, ed. Patterson, D., Castle House.

Appendix A: Quality-of-Life Assessment (Simplified) Self-completed Questionnaire

GM   General Mobility

Which one of these statements best describes your situation?

1. I can move around indoors and outdoors on my own easily with no aids or help. ☐

2. I can move around indoors and outdoors on my own with a little difficulty but with no aids or help. ☐

3. I can get about indoors and outdoors on my own *but* I have to use a walking aid, e.g. stick, frame, crutch, wheelchair, etc. ☐

4. I can move around the house without anyone's help but I need someone's help to get outdoors. ☐

5. I spend nearly all my time confined to a chair (other than a wheelchair). ☐

6. I have to spend nearly all my time in bed. ☐

UA   Usual Activity

During the past week has your health affected any of the things you usually do (e.g. at work or study or at home)?

1.	Not at all	☐
2.	Slightly affected	☐
3.	Severely affected	☐
4.	Unable to do usual activity at all	☐

Self-care

Do you need help with:

Washing yourself?	Yes	☐	No	☐
Dressing?	Yes	☐	No	☐
Eating or drinking?	Yes	☐	No	☐
Using the toilet?	Yes	☐	No	☐

Social and Personal Relationships

Does your state of health seriously affect any of the following?

Your social life?	Yes	☐	No	☐
Seeing friends or relatives?	Yes	☐	No	☐
Your hobbies or leisure activities?	Yes	☐	No	☐
Your sex life?	Yes	☐	No	☐

Distress

How much does your state of health distress you overall? Mark a cross on the line.

No distress
at all

Extreme
distress

├─────────────────────────────────┤

Appendix B: Conversion of (Simpified) Self-completed Questionnaire Responses to Rosser Categories

Disability

Coding: 'General Mobility' responses are already coded (GM) 1 to 6 in the questionnaire

Patients who are not conscious will simply be so recorded

'Self-care' responses are scored 1 for each 'Yes' response (possible range of scores is thus 0 to 4)

'Usual activities' responses are already coded (UA) 1 to 4 on the questionnaire

'Social and personal relationships' responses are scores 1 for each 'Yes' response (possible range of scores is thus 0 to 4)

Assignment rules

In the table below, first move to the appropriate *column*, using the 'General Mobility' response (or 'not conscious'). For GM4 to GM6 and for 'not conscious', no further information is required, the Rosser disability categories being V, VI, VIII and VIII respectively.

For GM1 to GM3, start with the 'usual activity' response. If UA = 1 (i.e. not affected) one of the first 3 rows will be relevant. If UA = 2 (i.e. slightly affected) one of the next 2 rows will be relevant. If UA = 3 or UA = 4, the Rosser disability category will be IV and V respectively.

For the first 5 rows the scores on Self-care and Social and Personal Relationships will be relevant, as indicated in the table.

Table for assigning respondents to Rosser disability categories

Other responses \ General mobility	1	2	3	4	5	6	Not conscious
UA = 1 SC = 0 *and* SP =0	I	II	III				
UA = 1 SC = 1 or 2 *or* SP 1 or 2	II	II	III				
UA = 1 SC = 3 or 4 *or* SP 3 or 4	III	III	IV	V	VI	VII	VIII
UA = 2 *BUT* SC < 3 *AND* SP < 3	III	III	III				
UA = 2 SC ≥ 3 *OR* SP≥ 3	III	III	IV				
UA = 3	IV	IV	IV				
UA = 4	V	V	V				

Distress

Coding: Measure position of cross on the 10 cm visual analogue scale in mm, with 0 at left end and 100 mm at right end. Treat this as the distress 'score'.

Assignment rules

Score	Rosser Category
≤10	A
>10 but ≤50	B
>50 but ≤90	C
>90	D

Measuring Health: A Practical Approach
Edited by G. Teeling Smith
© 1988 John Wiley & Sons Ltd

12

Implications for Clinical Practice

Colin Roberts
University of Wales College of Medicine, Cardiff

Early Applications of the Measurement of Health to Medical Practice

Measurement of health, which is the cornerstone of epidemiology, first came to prominence in 1662 when John Graunt showed that by counting deaths (the weekly bills of mortality) and births (from parish registers), disease entities (e.g. mortality from plague) and other health characteristics (e.g. infant mortality) could be symbolized in terms of public as distinct from individual health. This innovation, which simply provided numerical information on health by counting the number of persons with a given disease attribute, was a radical departure from earlier medical practice which had largely confined itself to a clinical account of the diagnosis and treatment of individual patients.

The opportunity to measure the health of populations in this way enabled certain objectives to be met which could not be achieved by traditional clinical investigation of the patient at the bedside, in the laboratory, or in the post-mortem room. Counting deaths and comparing them between populations provided information about the magnitude and deployment of health problems between different communities at one point in time and within the same community over a period of time. It thus provided an estimate of the size and distribution of existing health problems and also a baseline against which future health practices and any consequent social legislation could be judged.

There is good reason for regarding John Graunt as the father of health care planning for his bills of mortality were the forerunner of the official registration of births and deaths which was established in the United Kingdom in 1837. Today this information, which is incorporated into the standardized mortality ratio, plays a major part in determining the allocation of resources between regional and district health authorities in England and Wales (DHSS, 1976a).

The epidemiological measurement of health also provided a means by which the relationship between health and environment could be examined and set the stage for a wide range of investigations into disease aetiology. The aetiology fruits of Graunt's pioneering were first born in 1855 when John Snow published the first of his classic observations in the cholera outbreak in London. During the last half of the nineteenth and the first half of the twentieth century and, with the exception of the avitaminoses (Goldberger *et al.*, 1920) and the occupational cancers (e.g. luminizers' sarcoma—Martland, 1931, cancer of the bladder arising in rubber workers—Lueunberger, 1912) aetiological studies based on measuring the health of populations were largely concerned with infectious disease control. By the 1940s the problem of infectious disease had declined substantially and doctors were turning their attention to the investigation of chronic diseases such as cancer, ischaemic heart disease and congenital malformations. Because these were of much longer duration they required a much longer research commitment than did the aetiological investigations of infectious disease. This constraint tended to discourage clinicians, who were anxious to spend most of their time with patients, and the need arose for a new type of doctor who was prepared to devote his or her career to the aetiology and prevention of chronic disease. The consequent emergence of doctors, who were not practising clinicians, and who saw this as their lifetimes' work in medicine (e.g. CASE, Cochrane, Lowe and Stocks to mention but a few), marked the beginning of the development of clinical epidemiology as a discipline as distinct from its application as a method of controlling infectious disease.

From the 1940s onwards increasing use was made of the fact that, occasionally, epidemiological measurement of health could be used to study disease aetiology by experimental exposure of a population to a suspected cause. The success of this approach in helping to clarify, for example, the aetiology of dental caries (Arnold *et al.*, 1956) and retrolental fibroplasia (Kinsey and Hemphill, 1955) coincided with an interest in its possible application to studies of the effectiveness of medicine interventions. Early interventions were mostly controlled trials of vaccines and therapeutic agents. The last twenty years have seen this application widened to include complex clinical procedures such as intensive care for acute myocardial infarction (Mather *et al.*, 1971); technical diagnostic procedures in haematology, biochemistry and radiology; and mass population screening procedures for hypertension (D'Souza *et al.*, 1976) and breast cancer (Shapiro, 1982). It has also been suggested that experimental epidemiology should be used to examine the effectiveness of physiotherapy and psychotherapy (Cochrane, 1972) and speech therapy (Hopkins, 1975). One study even used this technique to examine the effectiveness of primary health care physicians by comparing them with nurse practitioners (Spitzer *et al.*, 1974).

The development of techniques which allow experimental epidemiology to be used to study the value of any activity induced upon a patient by any health care professional, owes much to the pioneering work of Professor A. L. Cochrane, the first director of the Medical Research Council's Epidemiology Unit in Cardiff. His important monograph *Effectiveness and Efficiency* (1972) has made Cochrane a legend in his own lifetime and his compelling argument for the importance of determining which of a variety of treatments for the same condition is the most effective, so that a rational therapeutic choice can be made, has now gained general acceptance as a method of scientific enquiry. However, while there may be general acceptance of the intellectual logic of Cochrane's thesis, there is little evidence that the results of such enquiries have, as yet had a substantial influence on clinical practice or any discernible impact on the development of health policy.

Why the Measurement of Health Will Influence Clinical Practice

Measurement of health, of itself, has no direct implications for the medical profession. However, as a process it enables certain objectives to be achieved which would previously have been unattainable. This derives from two important features which characterize the process itself. Firstly, it enables the impact of a particular disease on a community at a given point of time to be measured. Secondly, and perhaps even more importantly, by providing a means by which the impact of surgical, medical or social interventions on the prior health of recipients can be measured, it allows the effectiveness of specific health care interventions to be judged.

The effectiveness of a clinical intervention can be expressed as the frequency with which agreed health outcomes are achieved per 100 interventions. Assigning a cost to the intervention and knowing its effectiveness enables the cost of achieving the outcome (the outcome cost) to be calculated. This allows judgements about the worth and affordability of the intervention (see p. 258) to be made by the patient, in circumstances which the patient pays the doctor directly for services rendered (an open-market system), or by managers and planners of insurance-based systems whether they are privately funded (e.g. BUPA) or state funded (e.g. the NHS). For a further consideration of outcome costs and their calculation see Charny *et al.* (1986) and Charny and Farrow (1986), and of the distinction between open-market and insurance-based systems of health care see Roberts (1982), Charny and Farrow (1986) and Charny (1987).

The Demystification of Clinical Judgement

The vocabulary and the language used in judging the effectivess of diagnostic and therapeutic intervention has been, until recently, almost exclusively clinical and disease-based. For example, cancer treatment has traditionally been evaluated in terms of the radiological and pathological examination, the response of the tumour to treatment and subsequent adverse effects. Evaluation of diagnostic and therapeutic measures in, for example, hormonal and gastro-intestinal diseases is very dependent upon the results of laboratory investigation. The language of clinical and laboratory investigation is invariably disease- and pathology-specific—a language over which the medical profession has a substantial monopoly.

Broadening the measurement of health from a narrow disease-orientated base to include objective and functional measures of health, which can be referred to collectively as quality of life indicators, will have important consequences. The expression of outcomes of health care in terms of health as opposed to changes in disease states, by invoking a language which non-medical professionals and the lay public can also understand, will effectively break the monopoly of the medical profession in judging the effectiveness of its interventions. A wider constituency will now be able to sit in judgement on the benefits and costs of a particular health care intervention and the process of judging the worth of health care activities will therefore become more democratic. The demystification of the language of the clinical care and the democratization of health service management and policy-making that is likely to flow from it will have implications for the clinical management of patients and for the role of doctors as architects of health policy.

Measuring the Effectiveness and Efficiency of Health Care

Measurement of health is concerned with the study of health outcomes rather than the processes of medical intervention; that is with effectiveness rather than efficiency. Efficiency is concerned with increasing the number of interventions per unit cost or reducing the cost per intervention. At present efficiency studies are popular with politicians and health service managers because they require no value judgement about the worth and affordability of the intervention under scrutiny. A further reason for their popularity is that the findings of efficiency studies usually do not imply a significant change of role for the health care workers concerned and the implementation of any change consequent upon such findings is not like seriously to challenge management or its policies. Unfortunately the enthusiastic scrutiny, in the name of efficiency of the processes of, for example, waiting lists in the hospital sector, may be serving to divert attention form the fact that the objectives of these activities, and of the services which have developed to provide them, have yet to be publicly discussed and professionally agreed. Health measurement and cost utility analysis could change this situation quite dramatically.

There is good reason for believing that contemporary health care evaluation, and within this the important science of measurement of health, has substantially ante-dated the development of a conceptual and political framework within which it can be usefully applied. An immediate objective must therefore be to publicize the important role that health measurement has to play in the future planning and management of health services. Outcome studies using a change in health status as a criterion of performance will permit not only the best buy to be selected from a range of diagnostic and therapeutic options for the same problem but will also allow decisions to be made about the worth and affordability of a wide range of specific clinical and health care activities. Such information can be expected to have a major influence on future health planning and important implications for clinicians and other health care professionals. Implementing policy decisions derived from cost utility studies based on the measurement of health outcomes will therefore pose major challenges for policy-makers and for management.

The Likely Consequences of Combining Health Status Assessment with Cost Analysis

The expression, in a common form, of the health outcomes and costs of a variety of clinical activities, for example as a cost per quality life-year achieved, enables a direct comparison of the worth and affordability of different medical interventions. Furthermore, because the language of this comparison is no longer exclusively clinical, it will properly place the debate about the worth of specific health services in the arena of social policy rather than clinical judgement and as such is a matter to be decided by the public and politicians rather than by the medical profession.

A dramatic illustration of this potential for social change was seen recently in a British television programme (Yorkshire TV, 1987). A studio audience was invited to 'find out what it is like to play at being a doctor and choose which of two real patients should receive life saving treatment' A consultant physician and his patient—young mother suffering from renal failure—were introduced to the studio audience, who were then informed that the patient would die unless renal dialysis was made available. The consultant then described his patient's prognosis and expected quality of life if this treatment were to be provided. The audience was then introduced to an elderly woman who had been waiting for two years for a hip replacement and the consultant orthopaedic surgeon who was looking after her. The patient described the severity of the pain and the poor quality of life she experienced as a result of this condition. The orthopaedic surgeon then explained how simple and effective the operation was and how it could be expected to give his patient at least eight years of good-quality and pain-free life. The compère then told the studio audience that eight years of renal dialysis would cost £137,000 and that the operation for hip replacement would cost £2600, and that 50 patients in need of hip replacement could each be given a further eight years of good-quality life at the cost of providing eight years renal dialysis for the young mother with renal failure. At this point, and after having reassured the studio audience, consisting of approximately 50 unselected lay members of the public, that the situation 'would never arise in practice', the compère then asked them to 'imagine they had to make a policy choice between the two services'. To everyone's surprise the audience voted, by a substantial majority, to recommend provision of services for hip replacement.

The author has also witnessed similar unexpected judgements during district and regional health authority policy meetings about the use of skull radiography in head injury and the development of spina bifida and cervical cancer screening programmes. In the discussions of each of the above, in cost utility terms, there was, on every occasion, a clear tendency for the policy view of non-medical participants, such as the chairmen and lay health authority and community health council members, to differ significantly from that of health care professionals who were also present. The former were much more prepared to consider the relative social worth of the service in question and were consequently more selective in their recommendations about who the recipients of the service should be and its overall level of provision. These experiences lead the author to believe that the public's voice in health planning and management is largely unheard at present and that it could be expected to differ importantly from the views of health care professionals not only on a wide range of tactical issues such as those described above but on crucial strategic matters such as the desirability of providing screening in a publicly funded health service; the role of the hospital outpatient service in the continuing care of chronic disease; the balance between care and cure, and within this the role of the community health services; and the proportion of total national expenditure on health care which should derive from private sources.

Clinical Management of the Individual Patient

The Changing Status of Clinical Opinion

Having made a clinical examination and arrived at a diagnosis, the clinician initiates an action which he or she believes will benefit the patient. This assumption is an hypothesis which should ideally be verified just like any other scientific hypothesis. Verification of 'clinical' hypotheses can be difficult, for the circumstances are not so readily open to experimental manipulation and ethical constraints influence the extent to which the well-being of patients can be modified in order to test the hypothesis. The interval between the action and the outcome can be much longer in medicine than in the physical sciences, and the endpoint not so easy to recognize. Clinicians are practitioners by nature, anxious to get on with the task of doing whatever they can to help the sick, and many have neither the temperament nor the inclination to participate in the painstaking collection of the sort of evidence necessary to validate hypotheses about the effectiveness of their actions. These are some of the more important influences that have raised clinical opinion to its present status. However, with respect to a great many clinical activities undertaken with the intention of benefiting the patient, the status acquired by clinical opinion as a final arbiter of the truth or otherwise of any hypothesis implying benefit is probably out of all proportion to its value. As Cochrane (1972) said 'the oldest and probably still the commonest form of evidence preferred is clinical opinion. This varies in value with the ability of the clinician and the width of his experience but its value must be rated low ... it could be described as the simplest (and worst) type of observational evidence'. For further discussion of why this should be so see Feinstein (1967) and Roberts (1977).

The decade which followed the publication of Cochrane's monograph saw a gradual change in the medical profession's view of the relative importance of evidence and opinion. In 1983 Hampton, a clinician, took up this theme and in an editorial in the *British Medical Journal*, 'The end of clinical freedom', he wrote:

> clinical freedom is dead and no one need regret it passing. Clinical freedom was the right—some believe the divine right—of doctors to do whatever in their opinion was best for their patients. In the days when investigation was non-existent and treatment as harmless as it was ineffective the doctor's opinion was all that there was, but now opinion is not good enough. If we do not have the resources to do all that is technically possible then medical care must be limited to what is a true value, and then the medical profession will have to set opinion aside.

By the mid 1980s there was good reason for believing that doctors, in their choice of a particular investigation or treatment, were being influenced, to a greater extent than ever before, by published scientific evidence about the clinical effectiveness of their proposed intervention. The science of measurement of health and of quality of life assessment provides the means by which much of this evidence can be acquired.

Using Measurement of Health to Study the Links between Clinical Activity and Outcome

While there are obviously many examples of effective medical practice, measurement of health studies of medical care has shown that the links between activity and health outcome are not as strong as is generally supposed (Cochrane,

1972); McKeown and Lowe, 1974; McKeown, 1976; Newhouse and Friedlander, 1979; Royal Commission on the NHS, 1979; Brook *et al.*, 1984). There is little or no evidence at present to support the contention that clinicians who are habitually using more resources are necessarily materially altering the medical condition of their patients, although this is not an easy subject to investigate (see Kurylo, 1976, for a review of the methodology in this field). A comparison of Sweden, the United States, and England and Wales showed no apparent relationship between resources spent on health care and crude measures of population health (Peterson *et al.*, 1967). Martin *et al*, (1974), studying input into the care of patients hospitalized with myocardial infarction in the United States over a thirty-year period, found that there was an accelerating increase of inputs over time but no significant changes in the duration of hospitalization or mortality in hospital.

Dyck *et al*. (1977) showed that an audit of hysterectomies in Saskatchewan resulted in a fall of hysterectomies deemed unjustified on peer criteria from 23.7 per cent in 1970 to 7.8 per cent in 1974 and the total number of hysterectomies in the province dropped by 32.8 per cent. This fall did not appear to be associated with any negative health effects. Hampton *et al*. (1975) showed considerable variations in diagnostic test-requesting behaviour between general physicians without any apparent benefit to the patient.

More recently, further evidence of a lack of a close connection between the consumption of health resources and outcome has been obtained from the Rand Health Insurance Study (Ware *et al.*, 1987). Wennberg and Gittelsohn (1973) found variations in *per capita* consumption of various health services in thirteen different service areas of Vermont despite similarity of the population in terms of rates of illness, income, racial and social background, insurance coverage and *per capita* physician contacts. In fact there is evidence that increasing intervention may result in ill health (Schimmel, 1964) and where estimates have been made for the prevalence of the iatrogenic illness generally the results tended to be rather high (e.g. Malleson, 1973). Lichter and Pflanz (1971) have directed attention to the fact that areas where appendicectomy rates are high may also experience high rates of deaths attributable to 'appendicitis' which may in part be side-effects of surgery performed on those with normal appendices.

Many studies have documented variations in all fields of medical practice. It is a common feature of such studies that the variations bear no apparent relationship to mortality and morbidity. Examples are surgery (Gittelsohn and Wennberg, 1977), biochemical and X-ray test usage (e.g. Ashley *et al.*, 1972); Rose *et al.*, 1972; Hall, 1976; Rees *et al* 1976; Abrams *et al.*, 1979; Royal College of Radiologists Working Party, 1979; Sandler,1979; Williams and Dixon, 1979; Royal College of Radiologists' Working Party, 1975), hospital referral rates (Practice Activity Analysis, (1978), hospital admission rates, prescribing patterns, length of stay (Clough, 1978; Klein, 1982; Office of Technology

Assessment, 1983; McPherson, 1984; Yates and Davidge, 1984) and accident and emergency usage (O'Grady *et al.*, 1985).

Using Cost Utility Analysis to Derive Guidelines for Improving the Effectivess and Efficiency of Clinical Practice

With respect to day-to-day clinical practice in hospital many investigators have been concerned with the over-use of tests, particularly routine pre-operative investigations which, when ordered without clinical indication, tend to be uninformative (Kaplan *et al.*, 1982; Rucker *et al.*, 1983), which have no practical influence on decision-making (Rabkin and Horn, 1983; Catchlove, 1979) or on health outcome (Royal College of Radiologists, 1979). Kapan *et al.* (1982) estimates that in their hospital, where over 8,000 procedures were performed annually, abandonment of routine pre-operative biochemical tests might result in one potential avoidable death in a hundred years.

Roberts *et al.* (1983) showed that by applying the Royal College of Radiologists' guidelines which had been derived from a multicentre study of pre-operative chest X-rays, a substantial reduction in the use of this investigation was achieved in two hospitals with no apparent increase in perioperative morbidity and mortality. A cost utility analysis based on the earlier study estimated that it would cost at least £1m to save the life of a male aged 25–50 without cancer or cardiovascular disease by the use of this procedure (Roberts, 1983). These findings paved the way for a multicentre introduction of the guidelines into five hospitals throughout England and Wales and reductions of up to 50 per cent in the use of this procedure were reported again without any apparent increase in perioperative morbidity or mortality (Fowkes *et al.*, 1986; Fowkes, 1986). The RCR guidelines based on a combination of peer review and cost utility analysis are now widely used throughout the United Kingdom.

In 1982 Brand *et al.* developed a guideline for selecting patients with injured extremities who need X-ray examination which reduced X-ray usage by 12 per cent for upper extremities and 19 per cent for lower extremities. Overall only one fracture in 287 was missed for which the treatment was nevertheless appropriate and the outcome satisfactory. The authors estimated the use of the guideline in the United States would reduce X-ray charges by $139m.

The Royal College of Radiologists' Working Party on the Effective Use of Diagnostic Radiology has also conducted multicentre cost utility analysis for the use of skull radiology in head injury. After making rather generous assumptions about the effectiveness of skull X-ray in drawing the clinicians attention to the presence of an otherwise asymptomatic intracranial haematoma, the authors concluded that this benefit was likely to occur no more than once per 15,000 X-rays at a cost of £138,000 per benefit achieved (Evans *et al.*, 1983). Furthermore, it should not be assumed that 'failure to achieve this benefit' would necessarily result in serious outcome when surveillance at home by relatives, assisted by a head injury guidance note, was available. A set of guidelines, derived from this work, was applied in one busy accident and emergency unit for nine months. Over this period the use of skull X-ray in head injury was halved with no apparent adverse effect on health outcomes (Fowkes *et al.*, 1984).

The Royal College of Radiologists' Working Party has now produced a booklet of guidelines for good radiological practice which covers approximately 95 per cent of all radiological units currently used in NHS hospitals. The implementation and evaluation of this booklet is now proceeding in a pilot health authority where all consultants and their junior medical staff (approximately 200 consultants and 380 juniors) who used the diagnostic radiological facilities of one large teaching hospital have accepted the guidelines as hospital policy for an initial twelve-month period (Roberts, 1987). The study will shortly be enlarged to involve three more centres in England and one in Scotland.

The impetus for guidelines of clinical practice has been accelerated by a worldwide trend towards insurance-based systems of health care and a growing awareness, made evident by measurement of health and cost utility studies in clinical practice, that the links between health service activity and outcome are not always as strong as generally supposed. In the past it has been the tradition for the clinician to order all the diagnostic procedures that conceivably might help to clarify what is wrong with the patient, or what course of treatment should be followed. This traditional view ignores the stubborn economic reality that resources are finite and that it is no longer possible to be both endlessly generous and continually fair. Making judgements about the need for, and value of, services now forms an important part of coping with this problem. Clinical practice has to strive to be as safe as possible and to produce a given benefit at a socially acceptable cost. Clinical guidelines are recommendations, preferably developed by clinicians themselves, which describe how and when individual clinical activities should be offered in order to achieve these objectives. Guidelines are usually based on the results of formal studies which are then endorsed and promoted by a wide constituency of clinicians with experience in that topic. Such guidelines aim to help clinicians in their investigation of individual patients. Increasingly they will be accorded prescriptive status and junior doctors especially will be expected to account for departure from them. This substantial change owes much to the development of the science of health measurement which permits careful scrutiny of both the effectiveness and the cost of clinical activities. Although very much in its infancy at present, this approach is likely, in the fullness of time, to have considerable implications for day-to-day clinical practice.

The implementation of guidelines such as those described above, to assist clinicians in their investigation of individual patients, is rapidly gaining momentum. This notwithstanding, the development and implementation of a set of national guidelines covering the major aspects of clinical practice will take many more years to achieve. This is partly because much of the essential cost utility information is not yet available, partly because of the belief in clinical freedom, partly because of the clinician's desire to obviate risk to his own patients, partly because of the clinician's resistance to management, and partly and also crucially because of fear of litigation. For a further discussion of these issues see 'Introducing guidelines into clinical practice' (Fowkes and Roberts, 1984) and 'Clinical guidelines—medical litigation and the current medical defence system' (Harvey and Roberts, 1987).

The Relation between Clinical Responsibility and Health Policy

Much of medical practice is concerned with using medical knowledge and health care resources to avoid the risk of mortality and morbidity. The risks are principally the sequelae associated with not being diagnosed or treated properly or both (or not being diagnosed or treated at all). Publicly funded health services undertake to ensure and assure society's health risk avoidance through the provision of adequate resources. Clinicians are the organization's principal agents in executing this task.

The practice of medicine in the twentieth century has grown progressively more dependent on specialized high-technology diagnostic procedures to extend the clinician's powers of observation. Procedures such as tissue microscopy, biochemical analysis of body fluids, radiography, computer tomography and radioimmunoassay offer the benefits of accuracy and objectivity and permit the elimination of small risks associated with failure to make a proper diagnosis. Such risk avoidance is achieved at a cost—for any one procedure it may be calculated by multiplying the cost of the diagnostic test by the incidence of the disease among those tested. The decision that an individual 'could possibly have a particular disease' and that there is a diagnostic procedure available which could confirm or refute this is the exercise of a judgement for which the clinician is responsible. The decision that, under these circumstances, a publicly funded health service, such as the National Health Service should underwrite the cost of avoiding the risk is matter of social (health) policy. Unlike clinical decisions, social policy decisions have to take account of financial and other social costs and the loss of opportunity to use the money on other activities associated with improving health.

Clinical Responsibility

In the United Kingdom advances in high-technology medicine have moved ahead of the development of a social policy to cope with the financial and social implications of this progress. Examples are whole-body scanning, transplant surgery, and screening for cancer of the breast and cervix. Much of the impetus for the rapid development of high-technology medicine comes from the

United States which, having a largely private sector system of health care, is not constrained by the social implications of such clinical progress to anything like the extent which applies in the UK. For example, Foltz and Kelsey (1978) suggested that the reason why a policy of annual cervical cytology tests for sexually active women had been widely recommended to women in the United States (in spite of equivocal epidemiological evidence) and not in Canada or Britain is because 'when funding for a screening programme is mainly public it is ... necessary to assist competing priorities in determinations of need' in a way which is not true of a private system. The British National Health Service has tended to cope with this problem by ignoring the distinction between who is responsible for making clinical judgements and who is responsible for deciding health policy. In the United Kingdom the medical profession still plays a major role in determining health policy at regional and at district level.

There is a growing unease amongst clinicians that increasingly many of their day-to-day decisions create an inner conflict between their desire to help the individual patient and their desire to contain costs in a sensible way. The medical profession has as yet paid insufficient attention to this issue. This is due in part to a lack of awareness of the financial implications that a publicly funded system of health care has for the treatment of individual patients. It is also due to the profession's mistaken belief that the matter is one that may be resolved in medical practice by the exercise of *ad hoc* clinical judgement. In reality it is for society, not doctors, to decide what level of risk avoidance it wishes to finance, for it is society, not the doctor or the individual patient, who pays the bill. No better example could be found of the distinction between health policy and clinical responsibility

Who Should Determine Health Policy?

At present doctors view their role as creators and shapers of policy decisions in the health service as well as technicians responsible for decisions in the care of individual patients, that is, they believe in the freedom of doctors to determine what they do as well as how they do it. There is now a growing awareness that a separation of these functions is crucial to the proper planning and management of health services but this will probably be resisted by the medical profession, who will view it as a loss of power and status. Nevertheless, the basis for decision-making in the health service must rest on deciding its function and purposes and in this lay members of the public have as much entitlement to a view as professionals working in the health service.

As long ago as 1969, in the introduction to the report by the Task Force on the Cost of Health Services in Canada, the following statement appeared: 'at some points in the health service there is a need for those concerned to arrive at a philosophical balance between highly expensive services for limited general application and facilities which can be used by greater numbers of people'. The example given was heart transplants in a major city vs the lack of any doctor at all in a rural town, but it might equally have been dialysis programmes or intensive-care units or screening programmes for cancer of the cervix which, while used by large numbers of people, may not benefit very many. The time must come when society will need formally and according to plan (as it does now informally and haphazardly) to deny expensive treatment to some individuals in order that less expensive facilities may be made available to a larger number. Clinicians, by training and instinct, are too deeply involved —and rightly so— with the care of individual patients to be able to make these decisions. It is the public, through the machinery of politics and government, who must decide the priorities and who (in principle) must decide where and how much of their money should be spent on specific items of medical care.

It is tempting to allow this conflict of interests to remain hidden and to accept continuing irrationality in the allocation of resources rather than to have to face explicitly the difficult issues raised. This might explain why, with regard to the National Health Service, successive British governments have been primarily concerned with processes rather than objectives; recent examples of this occupation with inputs and processes are to be found in *Priorities for Health and Personal Social Services in England* (DHSS, 1976) and *Health Care and its Costs* (DHSS, 1983). The failure, to date, to examine the objectives of the health service may result from the view, widely held in society, that clinical freedom is the freedom of doctors to set service objectives rather than their freedom to implement these objectives for individual patients in their care. This denial of the social policy nature of health service objective setting may have benefited politicians by distancing them from the results of the rationing which is inevitable when finite resources are applied to an infinite demand for health care. Measured against the resource implications of clinical freedom the savings achieved through more effective management of non-professional staff and support services are modest. However, the power of the medical profession is such that no government, and none of the management initiatives introduced to date, have addressed the fundamental problem of management in the health service, *viz.* the freedom of doctors to determine what they do as well as how they do it. The history of management in the National Health Service is one of concentrating on efficiency rather than effectiveness, on tactics rather than strategy, and on the least powerful of groups such as the domestic staff rather than the clinicians.

It is possible that the autonomy of doctors (expressed in terms of clinical freedom) is not a privilege wrested by them from an unwilling body politic but rather a contract which suits both the doctors and the political masters of the health service. It is undoubtedly more comfortable for society to deny that rationing is taking place and, however unreal this assertion may be, it is made possible by the very fragmentation of everyday decision-making in the National Health Service. Of all the barriers to the implementation of proper management and planning this will be the most difficult to overcome. For a more detailed discussion of this issue see Charny (1987).

The techniques of measurement of health and cost utility analysis which have emerged out of the conceptual frameworks developed by Kamofsky (1948), Cochrane (1972), Rosser and Watts (1972) and Williams (1983) are likely to be of major importance in helping to promote the social change which is so urgently required. Although the underlying assumption of rational man is clearly false, making explicit the consequences of the present organization of decision-making may be expected to encourage a more detailed examination of the possibility of moving to a more efficient organization than exists at present.

Worth and Affordability

While economic growth has slowed, causing governments in most countries to seek to control public expenditure more firmly than hitherto, the expectations of patients and professionals have risen and the capabilities of medical and information technology have increased. If, as seems likely, the opposing forces of contraction and expansion continue for the foreseeable future, every passing year will require sharper choices to be made concerning which publicly funded health services should be provided and better managerial mechanisms to translate the resulting decisions into action. The important difference between affordability and worth will have to be acknowledged; publicly funded health care systems, like individuals, may not be able to afford some services that are worthwhile (Roberts *et al.*, (1985).

There is an important distinction between worth and affordability which remains largely unrecognized. It is widely supposed that if an economic analysis shows that the benefits of the service exceed its costs failure to fund it is irrational and inefficient. It has been shown by means of a simplified model of health care (Charny and Roberts, 1986) that although an excess of benefits over costs is a necessary precondition for providing a health service it is by no means sufficient. If society is to make the best use of its resources in health care, worthwhile services—those which make a social 'profit'—must be compared with other such services. Since the resources available to any publicly funded health care system will always be limited it is likely that not all services whose benefits exceed their cost can be afforded, because the budget has already been committed to those worthwhile services which yield higher benefits per unit cost. A decision that a publicly funded health service cannot afford a particular service does not, of course, imply an adverse judgement of its clinical worth. Unfortunately, clinical worth (effectiveness) is now only one of three dimensions which have to be considered before deciding whether an intervention can be afforded. The other two are the risk of the outcome to be avoided in the population at large and the cost of the intervention itself.

The implications for the clinician in all this are subtle but important. The worth of a particular clinical service is a judgement that the clinical and health benefits which can be achieved are worth the economic cost. The medical expert, from his personal knowledge of the suffering an individual might experience in the absence of a service, makes a vital contribution to this judgement, In contrast, the judgement that this particular service can be afforded out of public funds is determined by a social consideration of other health opportunities foregone. In other words, it is not a choice between life and death but between one person's life and the death of others—this is the price publicly funded health care systems pay for a fairer distribution of health care resources. Consider, for example, a typical district health authority policy decision. Recent savings have been made which could be used to expand either existing facilities for renal dialysis or hip replacement. The health authority should look at its clinical advisers to identify and quantify the health benefits that the two services can be expected to achieve and to its finance officers to calculate the relative cost of each service. No opinions are required at this stage for the information provided should be factual and capable of allowing its accuracy and validity to be independently verified. The scene is now set for the execution of a social policy decision. In the above example the allocation of resources to renal dialysis or hip replacement should be the responsibility of the lay members of the health authority and be based on their collective preference for one or the other. The financial and medical experts, having provided the information, should take no further part in this health policy decision. Unfortunately, this rarely happens at present because the language of the health policy debate is still too technical and specialized. The information derived from measurement of health and cost utility analysis, because it both simplifies and demystifies the language of clinical and health care performance, can be expected to play a crucial role in helping to achieve proper public involvement in the formulation of national and local health policy.

Conclusion

In his book Cochrane (1972) presented a compelling argument for the importance of determining scientifically which of a variety of treatments for the same condition is the most effective so that a rational therapeutic choice can be made. To this end he emphasized the importance of the randomzied controlled trial. There was much resistance to his message and although the objective was essentially a scientific rather than an economic one, it still took over a decade to gain the general acceptance it has today. In the present book, Teeling Smith and his co-contributors argue the importance of determining scientifically which of a variety of effective treatments for different conditions produces the greatest benefit per unit of cost. Should the need ever arise this method does at least offer a rational approach to the difficult task of deciding which types of condition a health service can afford to treat. Like Cochrane's earlier book, this present publication presents a message that is likely to face substantial resistance from some quarters because of its implications rather than its logic—all the more so because it concerns economic rationality rather than scientific propriety. The issue today, particularly for those health services that are publicly funded, is whether they can afford to provide the most effective treatment for every health need and for every patient with that need. Some may find the methodology, and more particularly the philosophy, unwelcome but there can be little doubt that by the early twenty-first century both will be widely accepted, by health care professionals and patients alike, as central features of health care planning.

The importance of understanding techniques for measuring health care and the effectiveness of therapy, and of cost utility analysis, is likely to be increasingly acknowledged in the syllabuses and professional examinations of a variety of health care profesional bodies. The subject is already of growing importance in medical undergraduate education and it is encouraging to find that its techniques and implications are well received by students. It is also likely to assume increasing prominence in the written papers for higher professional qualifications across a whole range of clinical specialties. All doctors, nurses and health care professionals serving on district and regional health authorities, and on their advisory committees, should have an understanding of the science of health measurement and its applications. Before long it is likely that short appreciation courses will be provided for all new lay members of regional and district health authorities and community health councils. It may not be going too far to suggest that this body of knowledge is as essential to the management and planning of the National Health Service as the Highway code is to the driving of a motor vehicle.

References

Abrams, H. L., Van Houten, F. X., Murphy, M. A. and Korngold, E. (1979). *Radiology*, **130**, 293–6.

Arnold, F. A., Dean, H. T., Jay, P. and Knutson, J. W. (1956). *Public Health Reports*, Washington, **71**, 652.

Ashley, J. S. A., Pasker, P. and Beresford, J. C. (1972) *Lancet* **i**, 890–2.

Brand, D. A. Frazier, W. H., Kohlhepp, W. C. *et al.* (1982). *New England Journal of Medicine*, **306**, 333–9.

Brook, R. H., Ware, J. E., Rogers, W. H. *et al.* (1984). The effect of coinsurance on the health of adults. Rand Report R-3055-HHS. Santa Monica, California: Rand Corporation.

Catchlove, B. R. (1979). *Medical Journal of Australia*, **2**, 107–8.

Charny, M. C. and Roberts, C. J. (1986). *Postgraduate Medical Journal*, **62**, 1107–11.

Charny, M. C. and Farrow, S. C. (1986). *Health Policy*, **6**, 363–72.

Charny, M. C., Farrow, S. C. and Roberts, C. J. (1986). *Community Medicine*, **8**, 199–205.

Charny, M. C. (1987). Risk targeting: the application of epidemiological data to problems of resource allocation in insurance based health care systems. PhD Thesis, University of Wales.

Clough, F. (1978). *Social Science & Medicine*, **12**, 219–228.

Cochrane, A. L. (1972). *Effectiveness and Efficiency. Random reflections on Health Services*. London: Nuffield Provincial Hospitals Trust.

Department of Health and Social Security (1976a). *Sharing Resources for Health in England: Report of the Resource Allocation Working Party*, London: HMSO.

Department of Health and Social Security (1976b). *Priorities for Health and Personal Social Services in England*, London: HMSO.

Department of Health and Social Security (1983). *Health Care and its costs: the Development of the National Health Service in England*, London: HMSO.

D'Souza, M. F., Swan, A. V. and Shannon, D. J. (1976). *Lancet*, **ii**, 1228–31.

Dyck, F. J., Murphy, F. A., Murphy, J. K. *et al.* (1977). *New England Journal of Medicine*, **296**, 1326–8.

Evans, K. T., Roberts, C. J. and Ennis, W. P. (1983). *British Medical Journal*, **287**, 1882–3.

Feinstein, A. R. (1967). *Clinical Judgement*, Baltimore: Williams and Wilkins.

Foltz, A. M. and Kelsey, J. L. (1978). *Milbank Memorial Fund Quarterly*, **56**, 426–62.

Fowkes, F. G. R. (1986) *Strategies for Changing the Use of Diagnostic Radiology*, London: Kings Fund.

Fowkes, F. G. R. and Roberts, C. J. (1984), *Effective Health Care*. **1**, 313–21.

Fowkes, F. G. R., Evans, R. C., Williams, L. A., Gelbach, S. H. *et al.* (1984). *Lancet*, **ii**, 795–6.

Fowkes, F. G. R., Davies, E. R., Evans, K. T. *et al.* (1986). *Lancet*, **i**, 367–70.

Gittelsohn, A. M. and Wennberg, J. E. (1977). On the incidence of tonsillectomy and other common surgical procedures. In Bunker, J. P., Barnes, B. A., Mosteller, F. (eds) *Costs, Risks and Benefits of Surgery*, New York: Oxford University Press.

Goldberger, J., Wheeler, G. A. and Sydenstricker, E. (1920). *Public Health Reports*, **35**, 648–58.

Hall, F. M. (1976). *Radiology*, **120**, 443–8.

Hampton, J. R. (1983). *British Medical Journal*, **287**, 1237–8.

Hampton, J. R., Harrison, M. J. G., Mitchell, J. R. A. *et al.* (1975). *British Medical Journal*, **ii**, 486–9.

Harvey, I. M. and Roberts, C. J. (1987). *Lancet*, **i**, 145–7.

Hopkins, A. (1975). *Health Trends*, **7**, 58–60.

Kamofsky, D. A. (1948). *Cancer*, November, 614–56.

Kaplan, E. B., Boeckman, A. S., Toizen, M. F. and Sheiner, L. B. (1982). *Anaesthesiology*, **57**, A445–7.

Kinsey, V. E. and Hemphill, F. M. (1955). *American Journal of Ophthalmology*, **40**, 166–79.

Klein, R. (1982). *Public Administration*, **60**, 385–407.

Kurylo, L. L. (1976). *Hospital and Health Services Administration*, **21**, 73–89.

Lichtner, S. and Pflanz, M. (1971). *Medical Care*, **9**, 311–30.

Lueunberger, S. G. (1912). *Bietrage sur Klinischen Chirugie*, **80**, 208–17.

McKeown, T. (1976). *The Role of Medicine: Dream, Mirage, or Nemesis?* London: The Nuffield Provincial Hospitals Trust.

McKeown, T. amd Lowe C. R. (1974). *An Introduction to Social Medicine*, Oxford: Blackwell Scientific Publications.

McPherson, K. (1984). *British Medical Journal*, **288**. 1854–5.

Malleson, A. (1973). *Need your Doctor Be So Useless?* London: Allen and Unwin.

Martin, S. P., Donaldson, M. C., London, C. D. *et al.* (1974). *Annals of Internal Medicine.*, **81**, 289–93.

Martland, H. S. (1931). *American Journal of Cancer*, **15**, 2435–41.

Mather, H. G., Pearson, N. G., Read, K. L. Q. *et al.* (1971). *British Medical Journal*, **3**, 334–8.

Newhouse, J. P. and Friedlander, V. J. (1979). *Journal of Human Resources*, **15**, 200–18.

Office of Technology Assessment (1983). Variations in hospital length of stay: their relationship to health outcomes. Washington, DC: Office of Technology Assessment of the United States Congress. (Health Technology Case Study 24.)

O'Grady, K. F., Manning, W. G., Newhouse, J. P. and Brooke, R. H. (1985). *New England Journal of Medicine*, **313**. 484–90.

Peterson, O. L. *et al.* (1967). *Lancet*, **i**, 771–6.

Practice Activity Analysis (1978). *Journal of the Royal College of General Practitioners*, **211**, 251–3.

Rabkin, S. W. and Horne, J. M. (1983). *Canadian Medical Association Journal*, **128**, 146–7.

Rees, A. M., Roberts, C. J., Bligh, A. and Evans, K. T. (1976). *British Medical Journal*, **i**, 1333–5.

Roberts, C. J. (1977). Epidemiology for Clinicians, Pitman Medical, Tunbridge Wells.

Roberts, C. J. (1982). *British Medical Journal*, **285**, 751, 754–5.

Roberts, C. J. (1983). *Journal of Royal Society of Medicine*, **76**, 755–9.

Roberts, C. J., Fowkes, F. G. R., Ennis, W. P., Mitchell, M. W. (1983). *Lancet*, **ii**, 446–8.

Roberts, C. J. (1987). *Clinical Radiology*, **39**, 3–6.

Roberts, C. J., Farrow, S. C. and Charny, M. C. (1985). *Lancet* **i**, 89–91.

Rose, H, Abel-Smith, B. and Deacon, R. A. (1972). A case-study of the demand for laboratory investigation in one hospital group. Occasional papers on Social Administration, London: Bell & Sons.

Rosser, R. M. and Watts, V. C. (1972). *International Journal of Epidemiology*, **i**, 361–8.

Royal College of Radiologists' Working Party (1979). *Lancet*, **ii**, 82–6.

Royal College of Radiologists' Working Party (1985) *British Medical Journal*, **281**, 1325–8.

Royal Commission on the NHS (1979), Report of the Royal Commission on the NHS, Cmnd 7615, London: HMSO.

Rucker, L., Frye, E. B. and State, M. A. (1983). *Journal of the American Medical Association*, **250**, 3209–11.

Sandler, G. (1979). *British Medical Journal*, **ii**, 21–4.

Schimmel, E. M. (1964). *Annals of Internal Medicine*, **60**, 100–10.

Shapiro, S., Venet, V., Strax, P. *et al.* (1982). *Journal of National Cancer Institute*, **69**, 349–55.

Spitzer, W. O. Sackett, D. L. Sibley, J. C. *et al.* (1974). *New England Journal of Medicine*, **290**, 251–6.

Task Force on the Cost of Health Services in Canada (1969). Reports, Vol. 1, Summary, Ottawa: Department of National Health and Welfare.

Ware, J. E., Rogers, W. H., Davies, A. R. *et al.* (1987). *Lancet*, **i**, 1017–22.

Wennberg, J. E. and Gittelsohn, A. (1973). *Science*, **182**, 1102–08.

Williams, A. (1983). The economic role of Health Indicators. In *Measuring the Social Benefits of Medicine*, Proceedings of a meeting held at Brunel University. London: OHE Publication, 63–8.

Williams, B. T. and Dixon, R. A. (1979). *British Medical Journal*, **i**, 1313–5.

Yates, J. M. and Davidge, M. G. (1984). *British Medical Journal*, **288**, 1935–6.

Yorkshire Television (10 June 1987). *Where there's Life*

Index

accident and emergency usage
  variations 253
amantadine 90 (table), 91
analysis of variance (ANOVA) 127–30
  repeated measures 129
angina pectoris, clinician's estimate of
  outcome 232 (table)
anticholinergics 90 (table), 91
antihypertensive drugs 16
  side effects 12
appendicectomy 252
Arthritis Categorical Scale 176
assessment of interventions, doctor–
  patient discrepancies 9–11
auranofin 158–9, 160
  cost-effectiveness analysis 181–4
  QALY calculations 182–4
  quality of life measures,
    selection/implementation
    160–81
  adverse effects 167, 168 (table)
  analysis of composite scores 180–1
  beneficial effects 167–8
  controlled clinical trial 163–5
  frequency of administration 165,
    166 (table)
  global measures 176–7
  measures of function 172
  measures of pain 169–72
  National Institute of Mental
    Health Questionnaire 180
  number of patients 165–6
  outcome measures 162 (table),
    170–3 (table)
  Patient Utility Measurement Sert
    (PUMS) 177–9
  Quality of Well-Being
    Questionnaire 160–1, 173
    (table), 174, 175 (table), 183
    (table)

Rand General Health Perceptions
    Questionnaire 180
  traditional clinical measures 168–9
  utility measures 177–80
  Willingness to Pay Questionnaire
    177–80
avitaminosis 246

Barthel Index 33
benefit-risk equation 4
benzhexol 90 (table)
benzotropine 90 (table)
biochemical tests, variations in use 252
biperiden 90 (table)
breast cancer 10, 150–1 (table)
  chemotherapy post-surgery 118
  natural history 111
  scenarios 77–84, 85 (fig.)
bromocriptine 90 (table), 91

cancer
  assessment of treatment 109–55
    clinical trials 110
    design of quality of life clinical
      trial 124–5, 126 (figs)
    patient selection 115
    phase I 112, 114
    phase II 112–13, 114
    phase III 113–14
    Priestman and Baum's test 121
    randomization 115
    sample size 115
    treatment protocol 115
  natural history 111
  occupational 246
  patients 13–14, 140–1 (table), 148–9
    (table)
  see also individual cancers
cancer-related states, utilities for 48
    (footnote)

cancer therapy, quality of life studies 123
category method 61
category rating 27–8
chloramphenicol 4–5
choriocarcinoma 111
clinical freedom 251
clinical judgement 2
  demystification 248
  estimating outcomes by 230, 231 (table)
    angina pectoris 232 (table)
clinical opinion, changing status 250–1
clinical practice
  effectiveness/efficiency improvement, cost utility analysis 253–5
  implications 245–60; *see also* health measurement
clinical responsibility 255–6
clinical trials
  death of patient 130
  health measurement 16–18
clinical worth and affordability 258–9
Cochrane, Professor A.L. 247
code of Hammurabi 25
continuous ambulatory peritoneal dialysis, utilities for 48
coronary artery-bypass surgery, quality-adjusted life years 40
cost-benefit analysis 2, 47
cost-containment 4
cost-effectiveness evaluation 46, 160
cost-utility model 64
criterion validity 62
cross-cultural issues 19
cyclophosphamide 132
cytoxic therapy complications 10, 13

dental caries 246
description 25–6
disease 7–8
disease scales 194–8
doctor–patient discrepancies in assessment of interventions 9–11

European Organization for Research and Treatment of Cancer Psychological Group 122
equivalence technique 60

factor analysis 26
5-fluorouracil 132
folate antagonist 110
function/dysfunction continuum measurement 37
Functional Limitation Profile 11
Functional Living Index for Cancer (FLIC) 30, 123
Function Status Index 64

gastro-intestinal diseases, utilities for 64
General Health Rating Index 197 (table)
gold, injectable 157–8
Graunt, John 245, 246

haemodialysis, utilities for 48
haemolytic disease 64
head injury, utilities for 64
health 8–9
  definitions 7, 192–3
    WHO 3,7
Health Assessment Questionnaire (HAQ) 172–3
health care, measurement of effectiveness/efficiency 248–9
Health Index (Grogono and Woodgate) 33, 34 (table), 45–6
health indices, utility measurement 198–9
health measurement 45–65
  acceptability to patient 16
  applications 63–5
  clinical practice influenced by 247
  cost analysis and 249–50
  cross-cultural issues 18–19
  early applications to medical practice 245–7
  epidemiological 246–7
  equivalence technique 60
  in clinical care 12
    clinical trials 16–18
  instruments 15, 197 (table)
  judgement 48
  links between clinical activity and outcome 251–3
  rating scale 52–4
  relevance to medical condition/treatment 14
  reliability/validity of instruments 14–15

health measurement (*cont.*)
  sensitivity to changes implied by
      treatment 15–16
  Standard Gamble technique 54–7,
      61–2
  time trade-off technique *see* time
      trade-off technique
  types 11–12
  utility values 49–52
    identification of health states 49
    preparation of health state
        descriptions 49–51
    selection of subjects 51–2
    use 48–9, 52
    validity 60
  see also questionnaires
health policy determination 256–8
health profiles 5, 194–8
Health State Classification System
    34–5, 47–8, 51
heart disease treatment 191–20
  rehabilitation 193
heart transplantation 10, 195
  case study 199–210
Heisenberg Uncertainty Principle 116
Hodgkin's disease 111, 134
Hoehn and Yahr's staging for
    Parkinson's disease 107–8
hospital admission rates variations 252
hospital referral rates variations 252
household survey 64
hypertension 12, 148–9 (table)
  doctor–patient discrepancies 9–10

illness 8
  iatrogenic 252
Index of Wellbeing 64
indicators of hospital performance 64
irritable bowel syndrome 211–12
  assessment 212–13
  health status/clinical measures
      relationship 216
  Nottingham Health Profile 212–14
    methods 213–4
    objectives 213
    results 214, 215 (table), 216
        (table)
  treatment 212–23
    effects 217–18, 219–22 (figs)

Karnofsky Index 30–3, 120, 194–6
Kupfer–Detre System 229

laryngectomy 48 (footnote), 50
length of stay in hospital variations 252
leukaemia, acute lymphoblastic 110
levodopa 90 (table), 91, 95
longevity *vs* impairment of speech by
    cancer surgery 50
low back pain, doctor–patient
    discrepancies 10
luminizers' sarcoma 246
lung carcinoma 111, 142–3 (table),
    144–5 (table)
lymphoma, indolent 111

McGill Pain Questionnaire 169
McMaster Health Index Questionnaire
    (MHIQ) 35–6, 197 (table)
magnitude estimation 27
management applications 225–43
  choosing descriptive framework 227
  gathering descriptive data 228–33
  interpersonal comparisons 237–8
  quality of life *vs* quantity of life
      236–7
  relative valuations 233–6
melphelan 132
methixene 90 (table)
methotrexate 132
mortality 24–5
  changing pattern 3
morbidity 24–5
measurement, purpose of 9
multiattribute utility theory (MAUT)
    34–5, 73
  multiplicative utility factors 76
      (table)
multidimensional scaling 26
myocardial infarction 12, 252

National Hospice Study 122
National Institute of Mental Health
    Depression Questionnaire 180
National Kidney Foundation
    Classification 229
New York Heart Association
    Classification 194, 195–6
Nightingale, Florence 25
non-compliance 12–13
non-curative treatments, comparison of
    two 134
non-steroidal anti-inflammatory drugs
    157, 158

North-Western University Disability
  Scale 92, 103–5
Nottingham Health Profile (NPH)
  11–12, 15, 197 (table), 200–4,
  209–10
  cancer patients 13
  content/structure 201
  defect 29
  heart transplantation study 203–5
  irritable bowel syndrome, *see*
    irritable bowel syndrome
  Parkinson's disease 93–4, 98, 99 (fig.)

orphenadrine 90 (table)
Overall Health Ladder Scale 176

Pain Ladder Scale 169
Pain Line 169
paired comparisons 28
Parkinson's disease 89–108
  activities 95
  Bulpitt's questionnaire 93
  depression 95
  Hoelm and Yahr's staging 92–3
  North-Western University Disability
    Scale 92, 103–5
  Nottingham Health Report 93–4, 98,
    99 (fig.)
  objective tests 92
  quality of life 92–100
  Sickness Impact Profile 93, 96–100,
    101 (table)
    Dysfunction Scores 100, 101 (table)
  speech 95
  symptomatology 89–90
  treatment 90–2
  unemployment 95
  Webster Rating Scale 92, 105–7
  written communication 95
patient
  death during clinical trial 130
  individual, clinical management
    250–5
patient-rated health scores 95, 97 (fig.)
Patient Utility Measurement Sert
  (PUMS) 177–9, 182, 186, 187
perceived health status 10
pergolide 91
phenylketonuria screening programme
  50, 64
prescribed items not taken as
  directed/thrown away 12

prescribing patterns variation 252
procyclidine 90 (table)
Psychological General Well-Being
  Index 197 (table)

quality of life 4, 10, 116–35
  contemporary definition 118–24
    physical/occupational function
      118–19
    psychological state 119
    social interaction 119
    somatic sensation 119
  design of clinical trial 124–5, 126
    (figs)
  interpretation of trials 131–6
  measurement 17
    criteria 119–20
  Karnofsky Index 120–1
  parameter analysis 127–30
  paradoxical trial 132, 134 (fig.)
  patient orientated measures 120
  tabular overview 139–55
    Australian survey 154–5 (table)
    breast cancer 150–1 (table)
    Calman 150–1 (table), 152–3
      (table)
    cancer patients 140–1 (table),
      148–9 (table)
    clinical trials 152–3 (table)
    coronary artery bypass 146–7
      (table)
    coronary heart disease 144–5
      (table)
    developing measure for QL 146–7
      (table)
    dialysis patients 140–1 (table)
    elderly 142–3 (table), 146–7
      (table), 150–1 (table)
    GPs' QL and medical decision
      making 144–5 (table)
    graduate/students 140–1 (table)
    haemodialysis patients 144–5
      (table)
    hypertension 148–9 (table)
    Karnofsky 152–3 (table)
    lung cancer 142–3 (table), 144–5
      (table)
    many meanings, Q/L 146–7
      (table)
    mentally retarded 140–1 (table)
    neonates 148–9 (table)
    oesophageal carcinoma 150–1
      (table)

quality of life (*cont.*)
  tabular overview (*cont.*)
    post-angioplasty 140–1 (table)
    proctocolectomy with pelvic
        ileal reservoir 144–5 (table)
    renal disease, end stage 142–3
        (table)
    sickness impact profile 154–5
        (table)
    social factor and disease 146–7
        (table)
    30, 50, 70 years 152–4 (table)
  Zubrod scale 120
Quality Adjusted Life Years (QALYs)
    40, 199
Quality of Life Assessment (Simplified)
    Self-completed Questionnaire
    241–3
Quality of Life Equivalent Years
    (QUALYs) 47, 76, 117
Quality of Life Index 30, 31 (table),
    121–2
Quality of Well-Being Questionnaire
    (QWB) 160–1, 173 (table), 174,
    175 (table), 183 (table)
Quality of Well-Being Scale 37–8,
    197
questionnaires 10–11, 17–18
  Bulpitt's 93
  cancer patients 13
  coding/analysing 16
  quality of life 14
  see also specific questionnaires

radiotherapy 13
Rand Current Health Assessment 176
Rand General Health Perceptions
    Questionnaire 180
randomized controlled trials 18
renal dialysis 64, 249
renal failure, end stage, patients 48,
    143 (table)
renal transplantation, utilities for 48
retrolental fibroplasia 146
return to work 193
Rhesus disease 64
rheumatoid arthritis treatment 157–88
  auranofin *see* auranofin
  disease-modifying agents 157–8
  non-steroidal anti-inflammatory drugs
    157, 158
Rhode Island Health Services Research
    161–3

Rosser's classification of illness states
    38–40, 228 (table), 228–9, 230–6
    passim
  valuation matrix 234 (table)
Royal College of Radiologists' Working
    Party 253–4
rubber workers' cancer of bladder 246

scaling method selecting 28–40
scaling techniques 27–8
scientific method 116
selegiline 90 (table), 91–2
self-assessment 14, 17
sickness 8
Sickness Impact Profile (SIP) 11, 36,
    197 (table), 198
  heart disease 198
  heart transplantation 198
  Parkinson's disease 93, 96–100, 101
    (table)
skin cancer 13
Snow, John 246
socio-medical data 10
Standard Gamble techniques 54–7,
    61–2. 179
surgery, variations in 252

Teeling-Smith Risk-Benefit
    Matrix 4
television programme 249–50
testicular tumours 111
therapeutic nihilism 135
time trade-off technique 34, 57–60,
    61–3, 69–85
  North American Development 71–6
    multiattribute classification 73–6,
    76 (Table)
    scenarios 71–3
  UK application 76–84
    characteristics of subjects 79
        (table)
    choice of subjects 78
    comparison with other values
        82–4
    construction of scenarios 77
    interview 77–8
    results 79–82
Toronto Activities of Daily Living
    Questionnaire 172
  Patient Utility Measurement Set
    167–8

Torrance's Health State Classification
　34–5, 47–8
treatment for different diseases,
　comparison 135
tuberculosis 2, 64
　screening 64

unemployment 3
Uniscale 122, 123
utilities 47, 64

valuation 26–7
very-low-birth-weight babies, neonatal
　intensive care 64

Webster Rating Scale 92, 105–7
well-being 10
willingness to pay 46–7
Willingness to Pay Questionnaire
　179–80
willingness to receive 47
World Health Organization, definition
　of health 3, 7

X-ray
　estimation of tumour size 115
　variations in use 252

Zubrod scale 120

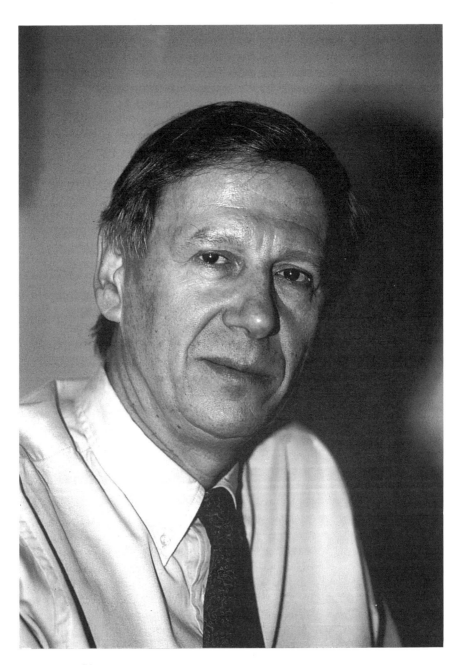

Anthony Giddens
Source: J.S. Library International